a/08

D0507102

HYPOCHONDRIAC'S
Pocket Guide to Horrible Diseases
You Probably Already Have

This is a work of humor. The diseases and the information on them are real, but some facts may have been omitted because they were boring or to make room for gratuitous profanity. This is not to be used as a medical text.

Published by Bloomsbury Publishing, New York and London
Distributed to the trade by Holtzbrinck Publishers

All papers used by Bloomsbury Publishing are natural, recyclable products made from wood grown in well-managed forests. The manufacturing processes conform to the environmental regulations of the country of origin —

Library of Congress Cataloging-in-Publication Data

DiClaudio, Dennis.
The hypochondriac's pocket guide to horrible diseases you probably already have / Dennis DiClaudio.—1st U.S. ed.
p. cm.
ISBN-13: 978-1-59691-061-4
ISBN-10: 1-59691-061-5
1. Hypochondria—Humor. 2. Hypochondria—Popular works. I. Title.

RC552.H8D53 2005
616.85'25—dc22
2005053014

ISBN 1-59691-061-5
ISBN-13 78-1-59691-061-4

First U.S. Edition 2006

10 9 8 7 6 5 4 3 2 1

Printed in Singapore by Tien Wah Press

THE

HYPOCHONDRIAC'S
Pocket Guide to Horrible Diseases
You Probably Already Have

DENNIS DICLAUDIO

BLOOMSBURY

CONTENTS

PARASITIC

TOXIC & FUNGAL

VIRAL & PRIONIC

INTRODUCTION

As we go about our daily lives—ordering a fourth round of mojitos, waiting in line at the supermarket to pay for our hummus, delicately hanging our photographs of tropical fish—there are a staggering number of things trying to get inside our bodies. Viruses, bacteria, worms, insects, bloodsucking fish. These things are hungry to enter our warmth and feed from our flesh, to multiply, to overtake our biological functions. And our immune systems cannot keep them all at bay. Some will get through, storm the gates, and ravage our fragile constitutions. And even as we are under siege from these intruders, we are being attacked from the inside as well. Organs faltering, neurotransmitters in the brain misfiring, long-dormant and mischievous genes sparking to life. It seems miraculous that any of us have lasted this long.

There are thousands upon thousands of diseases known to man. Medical texts on dusty library shelves are packed full with them. In writing *The Hypochondriac's Pocket Guide to Horrible Diseases You Probably Already Have*, I wasn't concerned with the huge majority of those diseases. After a great deal of research, I decided to settle upon a simple forty-five. The forty-five diseases included here are some of the worst, the deadliest, the strangest, the most repulsive, the most unpleasant maladies—all of them 100 percent genuine—that currently exist out there, waiting for you.

This book, however, was not intended to serve as a definitive resource for the included diseases. If, after careful self-diagnosis based upon your apparent symptoms, you come to the conclusion that you have Marburg hemorrhagic fever or cerebral sparganosis, get a second opinion. Seek the advice of neighbors and coworkers, the guy who sells imported salami to the guy who runs the corner delicatessen. Submit yourself to the capable minds of an Internet message board. As a last resort, you may want to consider talking to a qualified physician. But don't begin medicating or amputating yourself based upon the information contained herein. I, the author, am not a doctor. I am one of you—cowering, anxious, obsessively washing his hands. There are better authorities on these matters. Find them.

If you should find that you do indeed have one of the diseases included in these pages, please understand that it is not my intention to make light of your terrible situation.

You've got it hard enough as it is.

Please enjoy these horrible diseases, and may God have mercy on your soul.

—*Dennis J. DiClaudio, Jr., B.A.*

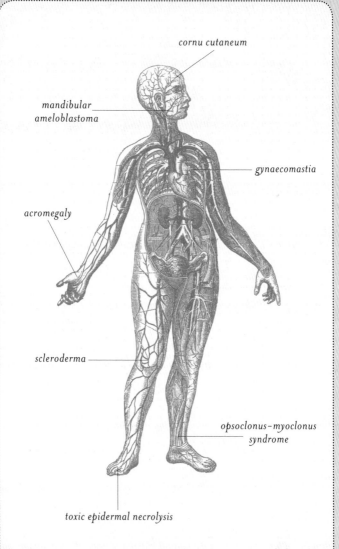

cornu cutaneum

mandibular
ameloblastoma

gynaecomastia

acromegaly

scleroderma

opsoclonus–myoclonus
syndrome

toxic epidermal necrolysis

AUTOIMMUNE

In which an overachieving immune system causes excess growth in parts of your body that were better left alone.

ACROMEGALY (ALSO GIGANTISM)

In which excess growth hormones make it necessary for you to keep buying new hats, gloves, and shoes.

SYMPTOMS

- enlarged hands and feet
- enlarged facial features
- spreading of teeth
- enlarged tongue
- swelling
- arthritis
- back pain
- curved spine
- tingling sensations
- numbness
- thick skin
- oily skin
- acne
- breathing problems
- fatigue
- headaches
- vision loss
- blindness
- change in menstrual cycle
- reduced sex drive
- impotence

DIAGNOSIS

It's funny how your body changes in very subtle ways, day by day, so that you never really notice it. You look at your reflection in the mirror and it seems a reasonable enough facsimile to the person you saw staring back at you yesterday, but in reality it's slightly different. Time takes its

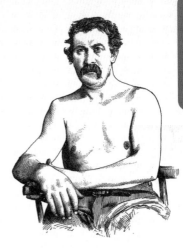

toll, not in great leaps, but in small, measured steps. You have a few less hairs. The wrinkles are deepening beneath your eyes. Your wedding band digs tighter into your finger. Your skull grows wider, your forehead more sloped. Gaps form between your teeth. And your jaw isn't supposed to protrude from your face quite so prominently, is it? One day, you meet an old friend on the street, and she says, "Holy shit! Why is your head so big?" It's all a part of getting old. Well, getting old and having an acute case of *acromegaly* (ak"-ro-meg'-ah-le).

The word itself is derived from Greek: *akro,* meaning "ends" or "extremities," and *megas,* meaning "large" or "super humongous." The effects of the disease, caused by an excess of growth hormones (brought on most often by a tumor growing on your pituitary gland), usually become apparent during adulthood, manifested as abnormally large hands and feet, but it can also give you a big nose, thick lips, a sloping forehead, and general facial disfigurement so that you end up looking kind of like folk-rock musician Neil Young.

And, yes, it can affect your penis as well.

PROGNOSIS

It will be much easier to bar chords on your guitar. With that and the penis enlargement, you might think that acromegaly isn't so horrible as horrible diseases go. There are some downsides. The growth hormones will also affect the organs, which can lead to heart disease, high blood pressure, heart rhythm disorders, diabetes, and colon cancer. Your chances of premature death will be increased 100 percent.

The disease is usually caused by a tumor of the pituitary gland, which is inside your skull, so all sorts of other problems may arise as it grows, squeezing itself against your brain and eyes. These may include headaches, vision loss, reduced sex drive, and impotence. So much for the penis thing.

PREVENTION

If you know a method for preventing tumors from growing inside your skull, then, by all means, use it.

TREATMENT

You can have the pituitary gland removed surgically. This will mean entering the skull through an incision in the nose and digging the tumor out. (Note: Please, do not attempt this on your own. Doctors are much more experienced with these things and have much better tools.)

Another option is drug therapy. Pegvisomant, octreotide, and bromocriptine can help to normalize the production of growth hormones in the body. But this can take years to have any effect, and even if it does, the disfigurement caused by overgrown bones is irreversible.

If neither option works, radiation therapy to the tumor may be necessary, but this may cause permanent loss of pituitary function, and you'll have to take hormone drugs for the rest of your life.

Of Note . . .

Andre Roussimoff, more commonly known as Andre the Giant or "The Eighth Wonder of the World," is probably the most famous victim of acromegaly. Diagnosed as a child, he made the most of it and became a professional wrestler, traveling the world and climbing into the ring wherever possible. Eventually asked to join the Worldwide Wrestling Federation (now WWE), he participated in six WrestleManias, at times held both Championship and Tag Team Championship belts, and defeated Big John Studd in the Body Slam Challenge of WrestleMania I. He also traded rhymes with Mandy Patinkin in *The Princess Bride*.

CORNU CUTANEUM
(ALSO CUTANEOUS HORN)

In which you grow a horn, not like a goat, but more like a rhinoceros.

SYMPTOMS

- itching
- tenderness
- skin discoloration
- skin growths
- warts
- a horn

DIAGNOSIS

Doesn't it always happen at the worst time? Your big job interview. The crucial first date with that cute girl from the gym. That indictment hearing for massive corporate fraud. You think you've got everything under control: the right suit, reservations at a trendy Thai restaurant, falsified expense accounts. Then you look in the mirror on the big day and—*boom*—you've grown a horn on your face.

Cornu cutaneum (kor'-nu ku-ta'-ne-um) always seems to know the most embarrassing times to show up, and since horns can sometimes grow to several inches in length, they're pretty hard to cover up. You can try to explain that it's just a hard, dense, pointy overgrowth of keratin (the

"Since horns can sometimes grow to several inches in length, they're pretty hard to cover up."

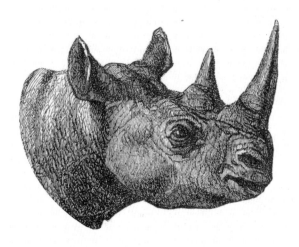

same material found in your hair and nails), probably the result of a minor skin tumor from being in the sun too long, but what does it matter? A horn is a horn.

CORNU CUTANEUM

PROGNOSIS

While you can grow a horn anywhere on your body, they tend to grow more often on your face and hands, areas that are more often exposed to the sun's radiation. The tumors that cause these horns are usually benign, but not always. So, while the horn is not technically a health risk, it may speak of a bigger problem.

PREVENTION

Stay out of the sun. Use lots of sunscreen. Keep away from radiation. If you notice any strange growths or discolorations on your skin, have them looked at by a dermatologist or zoologist.

"Keep away from radiation."

The horn is technically dead material, so it can be easily shaved off with a sterile razor blade. However, the cause of the horn will have to be dealt with. Depending on the type of tumor at the base of the horn, this may include such treatments as surgery, radiation therapy, or chemotherapy.

Of Note . . .

Your horn is not a true horn. The horns of most horned animals, such as a goat or cow, grow directly from the skull. Your horn is more similar to that of a rhinoceros, whose horn is also hardened keratin growing from the skin. So, if any "comedians" see your horn and decide to start calling you Goat Boy, you can quip back, "Hey, that's Rhino Boy to you."

GYNAECOMASTIA

In which men grow tits.

- tenderness of the breasts
- breasts

There are few things that the average man enjoys more than a nice firm pair of breasts. They hold a largely unequaled power to lift a man's spirits and lead him down dangerous but fun paths of temptation. It is quite a different matter, however, when the breasts are his. In fact, they tend to have the opposite effect. The thing about breasts is that they tend to look so much nicer on women.

To be clear, *gynaecomastia* (jin''-eh-ko-mas'-te-ah) is not your average case of flabby man-boobs, the last straw that gets you to finally sign up for membership at the gym. We're talking real C-cups (the kind of sweater satellites that more than a few women would eye cattily while sipping an appletini). These little friends are caused by an imbalance between the body's testosterone and estrogen levels. Too much estrogen in your system will cause your body to feminize itself. And then slowly—so slowly that you won't even notice it—the breast tissue will begin to increase, until you catch male coworkers in the street unbuttoning your button-down with their eyes.

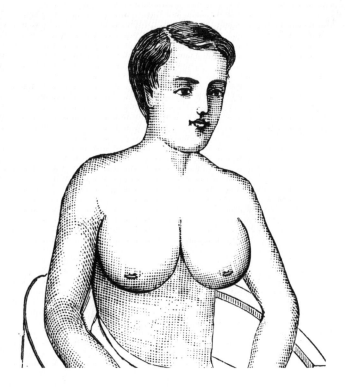

PROGNOSIS

You're going to have breasts, which really isn't that bad in the whole scheme of things. However, if your gynaecomastia is itself a symptom of another disease, such as cirrhosis of the liver, progressive spinobulbar muscular atrophy, or testicular cancer, that's another matter entirely.

Gynaecomastia may occur with other forms of feminization, such as water retention, softening of muscle tissue, fatty deposits in the hips, and an inability to answer direct questions in a concise manner.

PREVENTION

Many things have been known to cause increased levels of estrogen, but it should be noted that the most interesting (and annoying) one is the use of marijuana. Yes, smoking pot can cause breasts. So, you should maybe not smoke pot, or smoke less of it, or at the very least figure out a rationalization for why growing breasts isn't that bad after all. Other drugs thought to put you at risk for gynaecomastia include steroids, heroin, and antidepressants. And ask your girlfriend or wife to refrain from using vaginal creams that contain estrogen.

If your gynaecomastia has been caused by drug use, simply refraining from using that drug may cause the disease to work itself out, and your firm, full breasts will begin to recede. If not, lifelong hormone treatments may be needed. Or breast-reduction surgery should take care of the problem for good.

Many adolescent boys experience gynaecomastia to some degree during puberty. Usually not a gimongous rack, mind you, but noticeably perky protrusions of the T-shirt nonetheless. This is because God is always looking for new ways to torture adolescent boys. As they get older, God gets bored and moves on to some other poor kid, and the breasts should go away on their own. (If adolescence comes and goes and the breasts are still there, see above.)

Of Note . . .

The average breast-enlargement surgery can cost somewhere between $5,000 and $10,000. Gynaecomastia is free. So, before you take any steps to treat your gynaecomastia, just think of the money you're saving.

MANDIBULAR AMELOBLASTOMA
(ALSO ADAMANTINOMA, ODONTOGENIC TUMOR)

In which tumors on your jaw cause your face to become deformed.

SYMPTOMS

- pain
- loose teeth
- misalignment of teeth
- labored breathing
- ulcers
- facial swelling
- facial growths

DIAGNOSIS

Mandibular ameloblastoma (man-dib'-u-lar ah'-mel''-o-blas-to'-mah) isn't really that big of a deal. Not unless you're a person who's all hung up on the way your head is currently shaped. If you're so vain that you have a problem with giant bulbous growths disfiguring your jaw and pushing the teeth out of your mouth, then maybe mandibular ameloblastoma is kind of a big deal.

This disease occurs when tumors or cysts form on your jaw, growing at times to the size of a second head. The word *mandibular* refers specifically to the mandible, or lower jaw. This is where ameloblastomas most frequently occur, but they may also form around the upper jaw, sinuses, and eye sockets.

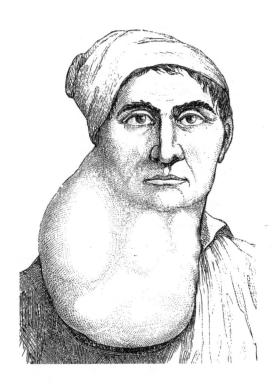

PROGNOSIS

Death is unlikely. But a lumpy, misshapen face is quite likely. It's a slow and persistent process, too, and most people don't realize they have the disease until it's too late.

Tumors and cysts grow in the tooth-bearing areas of the jaw. And then they keep growing. Teeth become loose and fall out. There is a visible swelling, and people say things like, "Hey, did you always have that rather large lump on the lower half of your face?" The result is large-scale jaw destruction and serious disfigurement.

PREVENTION

There is no real way to prevent mandibular ameloblastoma, because nobody really understands exactly why it occurs. It either happens to you, or it doesn't happen to you. Dental germs are probably at least partially responsible, so keeping good dental hygiene can't hurt.

The easiest, safest way to treat mandibular ameloblastoma is to have your entire jaw removed from your skull. This may sound like a bad idea, but try to keep an open mind. What do you really need your jaw for, besides eating, talking, and looking like a person who did not have his or her jaw removed? And with modern facial-reconstruction techniques, you will be able to almost look like a person who did not have his or her jaw removed. Not quite, but almost.

The other option is to have the tumors scraped away from your jaw. The upside of this is that you get to keep your jaw. The downside is that if even the tiniest bit of tumor is left behind, it can grow back, and then you'll probably have to go through the above option anyway.

Chemotherapy and radiotherapy have usually proven ineffective, though advances are being made.

Of Note . . .

Although most mandibular ameloblastoma tumors are benign, some are not. If you happen to get a malignant tumor, it can very easily spread to the rest of your body. And then won't you wish you'd had your jaw removed when you had the chance?

OPSOCLONUS–MYOCLONUS SYNDROME (ALSO KINSBOURNE SYNDROME, DANCING EYES/DANCING FEET)

In which your body attacks its own brain.

SYMPTOMS

- facial tics
- trembling
- shivering
- quivering
- shaking
- shimmying
- loss of coordination
- loss of balance
- loss of vision
- drooling
- confusion
- rage
- difficulty standing
- difficulty sitting
- difficulty speaking
- difficulty eating
- insomnia

DIAGNOSIS

You would think that your body's autoimmune system would be able to tell the difference between a virus that's infecting your body and your own brain. You would think. But that's not always the case, as evidenced by *opsoclonus-myoclonus syndrome* (op"-so-klo'-nus mi-o-klo'-nus). In this situation, your immune system sends out what can only be assumed to be very stupid antibodies to attack and destroy the infectious virus, except that the antibodies get confused and panicky and mistake your brain cells—usually the ones in the cerebellum, brainstem, and limbic system—for the virus. So they start killing your brain cells. Just slaughtering them by the millions. It's a total massacre.

Meanwhile, the work that the innocent brain would have been doing isn't getting done; there's no one manning the control panel, so everything goes crazy. Your hand-eye coordination deteriorates. Your eyes dart nervously around inside their sockets. Your muscles twitch. Standing up becomes a nearly impossible task. You can't think straight. You can't sleep. It's a disaster.

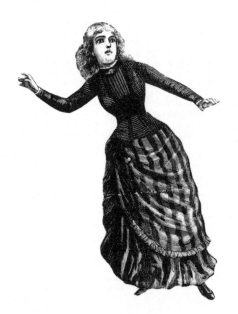

PROGNOSIS

It's going to be difficult for you to move around or see straight or, generally speaking, just do things. There will be a lot of jerking and trembling. These problems will increase when you try to do things. They will also increase when you become frustrated or agitated.

The good news is that opsoclonus-myoclonus syndrome is very rarely fatal. However, the viruses that cause opsoclonus-myoclonus syndrome, well, uh . . . sorry.

PREVENTION

A number of viruses, such as Epstein-Barr, coxsackie, and encephalitis (page 186), have been known to trigger opsoclonus-myoclonus syndrome. Try not to get any of them.

> "You can't think straight.
> You can't sleep.
> It's a disaster."

Azathioprine, an immunosuppressive agent, may be sent into your body to act as a sort of negotiator, to try to come to a peace accord with your immune system's B cells so that they may slow down the production of antibodies. If a peace accord is not possible, you may need to undergo immunoadsorption, a medical procedure through which the antibodies are forcibly removed from your body.

Hopefully, you'll be able to calm things down inside there quickly, or the damage to your brain may be permanent.

Of Note . . .

Opsoclonus-myoclonus syndrome can also be caused by certain tumors—not necessarily in your brain—which are genetically similar to brain cells. However, it is not yet understood how even incredibly stupid antibodies can confuse your brain, which almost always rests in the head, with a tumor as far away as your chest.

SCLERODERMA

*In which your skin and organs slowly harden and you
begin to resemble a human statue.*

SYMPTOMS

- numbness, pain, or
  discoloration in the
  extremities
- aches in the joints or
  bones
- sores over joints
- puffy hands or feet
- hardening of the skin

- skin discoloration
- difficulty swallowing
- dry mucous membranes
- fatigue
- high blood pressure
- weight loss
- heartburn

DIAGNOSIS

You can buy the finest European moisturizers. Rub yourself
with freshly picked aloe. You can take baths in extra-virgin
olive oil and pack your face with mud from the Dead Sea.
You can inject pure royal jelly from the hives of South
African bees directly into your pores, and it won't do you
any good.

Scleroderma (skle''-ro-der'-mah) is a chronic autoimmune
disease that causes hardening and tightening of the skin and

its connective tissue. The very name of the disease is Greek for "hard skin." It results from your body's immune system producing an excess of collagen in your body's tissues. This has the effect of hardening your skin over the course of a few years so that it becomes like toughened leather stretched tightly across your bones. Your joints seize up and your muscles shrink, so that movement is extremely difficult and painful. Your hands and feet grow into gnarled claws. The skin around your mouth, nose, and eyes stiffens your features into a disfigured grimace. Your invitations to very fancy parties diminish to almost nil.

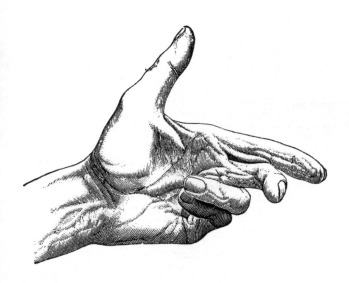

PROGNOSIS

Although its most obvious effects (i.e., hard and shiny skin, loss of mobility, disfigured grimace) are external, scleroderma also has a considerable effect on blood vessels and major organs. It can cause your intestinal tract to cease absorbing nutrients. Your lungs and heart may become scarred, leading to an inability to breathe properly and the onset of congestive heart failure. Of the ten thousand people who die from scleroderma each year, most die from these effects.

PREVENTION

Scleroderma is not contagious, but its causes are still unknown, so there's no way to best prevent it. If you do figure out a way to prevent it, please contact the Scleroderma Research Foundation in San Francisco, California (www.srfcure.org), as they will most certainly be happy to hear from you.

There is no cure for or way to stop the progressive effects of scleroderma, but there are many drugs that can help suppress its symptoms. These include COX-2 inhibitors, H-2 blockers, prokinetic agents, endothelin receptor antagonists, immunosuppressants, and aspirin (go figure).

> "Your invitations to very fancy parties diminish to almost nil."

Of Note . . .

Scleroderma was first documented by Dr. Carlo Curzio of Naples in 1754. He described his seventeen-year-old patient as having "an excessive hardness of her skin over all of her body, by which she found herself so bound and straightened that she could hardly move her limbs." He was unable to cure his patient, but he did create quite a name for himself and was invited to many very fancy parties (she, sadly, was not).

TOXIC EPIDERMAL NECROLYSIS (ALSO LYELL'S DISEASE)

In which your skin erupts in painful blisters and rashes and eventually peels off in sheets.

SYMPTOMS

- fatigue
- rash
- sores
- blisters
- bleeding
- fever
- cough
- sore throat
- muscle pain
- burning sensation
- sensitive skin
- scalded skin
- sensitivity to light
- skin peeling off in sheets
- pain
- pus
- crusted lips
- cracked lips
- bleeding lips
- loss of appetite
- hair loss
- dry eyes
- eye pain
- vision loss
- blindness

DIAGNOSIS

Like the stately Monarch caterpillar, spinning a silky cocoon around itself on the leaf of a milkweed plant, so you, too, have begun your change. The small red patches of rash on your face, neck, chest, and genitals are spreading, growing into one another and erupting in painful blisters. Your upper layer of skin is coming loose and sagging, with pockets of fluid oozing noticeably beneath it. And, as the caterpillar soon finds itself within its glistening waxy chrysalis, so you have found yourself encased in a complete layer of dead skin, with eyes peering outward from the confines of your necrotized shell. But, when this skin ruptures and comes peeling off in great swathes, you will not be emerging, with wings stretched skyward, but as a scalded, trembling, muculent figure, oozing pus and resembling nothing so much as the tenant of a burn victim's ward.

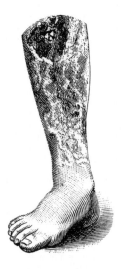

Although many questions about *toxic epidermal necrolysis* (tok'-sik ep"-i-der'-mal ne-krol'-i-sis) still puzzle doctors, it is generally believed that it occurs because of your body's inability to metabolize a drug (usually a prescribed drug, the kind that is, you know, supposed to make you feel better). The body deposits the unwanted drug in the outermost layer of skin and then wants nothing more to do with it.

TOXIC EPIDERMAL NECROLYSIS CONTINUED

PROGNOSIS

When toxic epidermal necrolysis occurs, it moves quickly. Within three or four days, you'll progress from simple flu-like symptoms to having rashes and blisters covering your body. Shortly after that, your top layer of skin peels right off.

You have about a 30 percent chance of dying, probably from widespread systemic infection due to the gigantic open sore where your top layer of skin used to be.

PREVENTION

There is no effective way to prevent toxic epidermal necrolysis. Though it is usually brought on by a negative reaction to a particular drug, there are at least a hundred drugs known to cause the disease—a few of the more likely ones are penicillin, sulfadiazine, and phenytoin—so it's hard to guess which one might bring on the disease. In certain cases, however, the cause of the disease is unknown. It just happens.

TREATMENT

There is no way to treat toxic epidermal necrolysis specifically.

You'll probably be admitted to a hospital's burn ward and be treated as a burn patient, with your body covered in antiseptics and wrapped in bandages, or possibly grafted with the skin of a cadaver, to stave off infections. Your fluid and electrolyte depletion will be carefully monitored and replacements administered. If doctors can determine the drug responsible for the negative reaction, its use should be terminated immediately.

Some doctors advocate the use of corticosteroids to control inflammation, but others disagree, as they suppress the immune system, leaving you open to infections. And corticosteroids are another drug known to cause toxic epidermal necrolysis.

With a few weeks of proper medical care, your body should heal enough for you to return to a relatively normal life. Expect lots of cool scars.

Of Note . . .

While lying in your intensive-care bed, flayed like a grape, with doctors and nurses poking and prodding at your exposed flesh, all because you took a drug that you probably shouldn't have been prescribed, you will be able to find some solace in the calming therapeutic buzz of the few dozen prosecuting attorneys that will almost certainly be hovering just outside your hospital-room door, waiting, waiting . . .

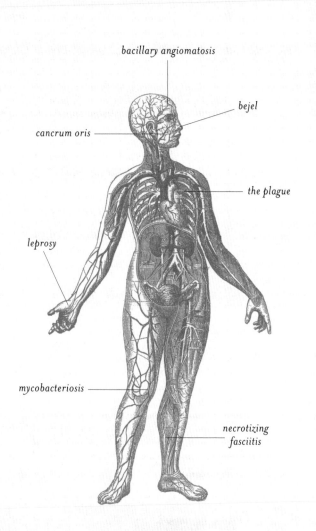

bacillary angiomatosis

bejel

cancrum oris

the plague

leprosy

mycobacteriosis

necrotizing
fasciitis

BACTERIAL

In which one of the many types of single–celled

microorganisms takes residence within you.

BACILLARY ANGIOMATOSIS
(ALSO BARTONELLOSIS, CAT SCRATCH FEVER,
CAT SCRATCH DISEASE)

In which your pet cat infects you with its bacterial infection.

SYMPTOMS

- fever
- headache
- muscle pain
- sore throat
- neck pain
- joint pain
- pimples
- sores
- bloody cysts
- fatigue

- loss of appetite
- weight loss
- anorexia
- nausea
- vomiting
- vision loss
- blindness
- convulsions
- coma

DIAGNOSIS

Oh my God! Kittens are so cute, aren't they? Yes, they certainly are. They are sooo cute! Don't you love it when they roll themselves up into itty-bitty little fuzzy balls on your lap and fall asleep? Isn't that adorable? Or when they lie on their backs with their soft fluffy bellies in the air and stretch their paws waaaaay up over their heads like a big kitty? Or how about when they pass on their *Bartonella henselae* (bar"-to-nel'-lah hen'-sah-lay) bacterial infections to you? And what about those pus-filled lesions that form at the point of infection on your skin? Pus-filled lesions are sooo cute!! But not as cute as the bloody cysts that follow once the bacteria has had time to settle into your system. Couldn't you just eat them up? Too bad you won't be able to see all this for much longer, since you're going blind.

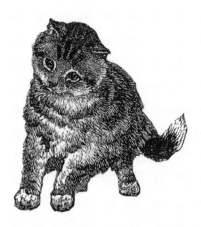

Bacillary angiomatosis (bas'-i-la"-re an"-je-o-mag-to'-sis) is almost exclusively passed on to people by a cat scratch or bite. Nearly 50 percent of all cats carry *Bartonella henselae* at some point in their lives, and that includes pet cats, usually while kittens, and especially if they're cute. Infection most frequently occurs because of a minor scratch or bite, often while playing with the kitten. It may also occur because of a simple lick, when your very cute cat is telling you that it loves you very much. It's very hard to tell if a cat is infected, as it usually only causes a slight fever in them that lasts a few days. Others may show no signs at all.

PROGNOSIS

The infection will usually first become apparent as a small pimple or sore at the point of the cat scratch or bite. After a few weeks, you may notice a swelling in your lymph nodes and some flu-like symptoms. Sometimes it ends there, fading away after a few months. Other times, however, more serious symptoms may arise, such as cysts on the skin and vision loss.

PREVENTION

Don't play rough with your cat. Don't play with your cat. Wear gloves while handling your cat. Send your cat outside to use "nature's bathroom," and then, when it mews at the back door trying to get back in, pretend you don't hear it until it gets bored and goes away.

Antibiotics such as erythromycin and tetracycline have proven effective against the disease, especially if it is caught early.

> "Kittens are so cute, aren't they?
>   Yes, they certainly are.
>   They are sooo cute!"

Of Note . . .

In the 1977 song "Cat Scratch Fever," Ted Nugent claims to have been infected with bacillary angiomatosis several times. However, the symptoms described in his song do not fully match up with the findings of medical research. Despite his claim that "it makes a grown man cry, cry," there is no evidence that the disease affects the tear ducts. It could be that Mr. Nugent was misdiagnosed and actually had melioidosis, an infectious bacterial disease that usually affects horses and goats.

BEJEL (ALSO ENDEMIC SYPHILIS)

In which you get syphilis simply by touching someone.

SYMPTOMS

- sore throat
- swollen lymph nodes
- oral or nasal ulcer
- blistering
- leg pain
- lesions
- lumps on skin
- tumor-like growths
- bone deformation

DIAGNOSIS

Everybody wants syphilis! But who wants to deal with all the sex involved in getting it? All that hassle. All that mess. Sweaty torsos and bodily fluids. There's got to be a better way . . .

Good news! You *don't* need to have sexual intercourse to contract one of the world's most popular social diseases. Now there's bejel!

Bejel (bej'-el) utilizes the innovative powers of *Treponema pallidum endemicum* (trep''-o-ne'-mah pal'-eh-dum en-dem'-eh-kum), a strain of the common syphilitic bacteria, to create a disease that is uncomfortable and disfiguring but does not need to be transferred through genital secretion. Bejel is transferable simply through direct or indirect bodily contact. Sure, bejel is most easily acquired from the open sores of an infected person, but you can also get it from a contaminated hand or eating utensil. It's just that easy!

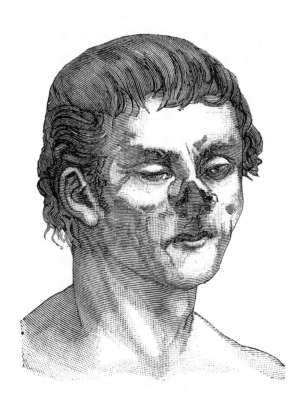

PROGNOSIS

Most likely, you won't die. But you may very well find yourself terribly deformed. You may die, though. It's definitely possible.

In the early stages of infection, ulcers will form in your mouth, throat, and nasal cavities. These give way to tumor-like growths. If left untreated, these may spread to your skull, cartilage, and skin, then begin eating away at your face.

PREVENTION

Don't touch anybody. Don't let anybody touch you. Don't shake hands. Don't high-five. Don't hug. Don't kiss. Don't let anybody reach over to wipe a piece of lint off your cheek. Don't support anybody in the crook of your arm. Don't eat with a fork that may have been used by somebody else. Don't take a sip of wine from the glass of an attractive and well-read person at a cocktail party. Don't go anywhere near any person who has an open sore, even if it's hidden beneath his or her clothes.

Bejel is curable with large doses of benzathine penicillin G injected directly and painfully into your muscle. Antibiotics, such as tetracycline and chloramphenicol, taken orally, have also been known to help. Of course, none of this will make your nose grow back, so try to have it treated in its early stages.

BACTERIAL

> "Don't touch anybody.
> Don't let anybody touch you.
> Don't shake hands.
> Don't high-five.
> Don't hug.
> Don't kiss."

Of Note . . .

Syphilis is also available in two other fun flavors, yaws and pinta, which are also infectious through bodily contact but are caused by different strains of the *Treponema pallidum* bacteria.

CANCRUM ORIS
(ALSO NOMA, GANGRENOUS STOMATITIS)

In which bacteria eats away at your face.

SYMPTOMS

- excessive salivation
- oral sores
- itching, swollen gums
- halitosis
- discoloration of the skin

DIAGNOSIS

The Greek word *nomein* serves as the etymological ancestor of the word *noma* (no'-mah), the common name for cancrum oris. *Nomein* means "to devour." Unfortunately, in the case of cancrum oris, the thing that is being devoured is your face.

Cancrum oris (kang'-krum o'-ris) is a sort of gangrene of the mouth's lining, beginning with painful ulcers, halitosis, and irritated gums. The sores spread quickly to the cheeks and bone as the active bacteria eats away at your mucous membranes, the tissue of your lips and facial skin dies, your teeth loosen, and a black patch of gangrenous rot grows across the affected area. Soon thereafter, the mutilated jaw is clearly visible through the ingurgitated wound. It's sort of like having a window in the side of your head with a fantastic view of your teeth.

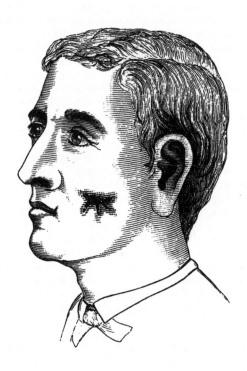

PROGNOSIS

Luckily for you, despite the fever, malaise, and tachycardia that often accompany the disease, fewer than 10 percent of people who contract cancrum oris actually die from it. Instead, they get to spend the rest of their lives with half a mouth.

If left untreated, cancrum oris can spread to the tonsils, nose, ears, scalp, and eyelids.

PREVENTION

Brush your teeth and eat well. Lack of cleanliness and a poor diet are major contributors to the contraction of cancrum oris. Also, if it's not too much of a bother, try not to use any anti-inflammatory or immunosuppressive drugs, like steroids or cyclophosphamide, which make you more susceptible to the disease.

Antibiotics can stop the disease's encroaching necrotic effects, but extensive reconstructive facial surgery will be necessary to make you look like anything approaching normal.

"It's sort of like having a window in the side of your head with a fantastic view of your teeth."

Of Note . . .

Cancrum oris is closely related to a disease called *noma pudendi*, which has a very similar progression but affects your genitals instead.

LEPROSY
(ALSO HANSEN'S DISEASE, LEPRA)

In which your hands and feet go numb and eventually fall off.

SYMPTOMS

- numbness
- tingling sensation
- swelling
- sores
- thickened skin
- congestion

- nosebleeds
- loss of vision
- blindness
- deformity
- loss of body parts

DIAGNOSIS

You'd think that after all these years many of the misplaced fears and naïve beliefs about *leprosy* (lep'-ro-se)—or as it has been more recently known, Hansen's disease—would have become extinct. Unfortunately, that's not the case. So, some things should be cleared up before going any further.

No, you cannot contract leprosy simply through the gaze of an infected person or by being in close proximity to one. You would have to touch an infected person or inhale some of his or her infected respiratory droplets, which are let loose in the air when he or she coughs.

No, victims of leprosy do not, for the most part, live in isolated colonies anymore. Now victims of leprosy are free to live and work wherever they please. There are a few thousand victims living in the United States today, and several hundred new cases are reported every year. In fact, one might be sitting next to you on the subway tomorrow.

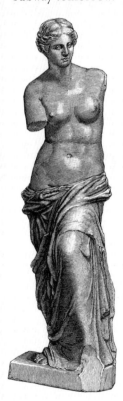

No, leprosy is not caused by the wrath of God. It is caused by the bacteria *Mycobacterium leprae* (mi"-ko-bak-tir'-e-um lep'-re), which enters the body through the mouth, nose, or skin and then progressively moves throughout the body and into the nervous system, causing thick, numb patches of skin, loss of sensation, and vision problems. God, really, has nothing to do with it.

No, leprosy does not cause your body parts to fall off. What a bunch of nonsense that is. It is the nerve damage—caused by leprosy and which leads to small wounds going unnoticed until they have grown gangrenous—that causes your body parts to grow disfigured and eventually fall off. Technically, it's not the leprosy.

PROGNOSIS

Usually, leprosy will first manifest as several patches of numb skin. These will most commonly occur on your extremities, such as your hands, feet, and testicles. First, the affected areas will lose the ability to distinguish extremes in temperature. Then, they will not sense light touching, then they will not sense pain, and finally they will not sense heavy pressure.

Your affected skin will grow pale and hard. Open sores will erupt. If these—or any other small injuries to the area—are not noticed and treated, they will become infected and begin to rot and eat into your bones. Eventually, body parts will begin coming off.

PREVENTION

Cleanliness is key. Always wash your hands thoroughly after shaking a coworker's gangrenous stump.

Also, do not incur the wrath of God (just in case).

"Always wash your hands thoroughly after shaking a coworker's gangrenous stump."

TREATMENT

Leprosy can be easily cured in its early stages through use of the antibacterial drugs dapsone, rifampicin, and clofazimine. If these don't work for some reason, you might want to try gorging yourself on the flesh of tortoises. There's no scientific backing for this treatment, but they used to do it in the Chagos Islands of the Indian Ocean, and supposedly it can taste pretty good if prepared correctly.

Of Note . . .

Leprosy is listed in the Guinness Book of World Records as the oldest known disease, having first been reported in Egypt in 1350 BCE. (Suck it, anthrax!)

MYCOBACTERIOSIS

(ALSO FISH-HANDLER'S DISEASE, SWIMMING-POOL GRANULOMA)

In which your pet fish infect you with their mycobacteria.

SYMPTOMS

- O inflammation
- O joint pain
- O lumps
- O rash
- O lesions

- O boils
- O ulcers
- O malaise
- O nausea
- O vomiting

DIAGNOSIS

The fish in your aquarium, just look at them. Malayan angels, black mollies, milk-spotted puffers, African scats. See the cold, dead look in their eyes? They're biding their time. Swimming back and forth. Back and forth. Waiting for the perfect opportunity. But they won't be obvious about it. They won't leap from their glass cage and undulate their way across the hardwood floor toward your cowering, crumpled form in the corner of the room. No. They have something much more insidious in mind.

With each crimple and curve of their sleek, burnished bodies, they are shedding thousands of mycobacteria into the stagnant water in which they live. They will slowly turn their small home into a festering cauldron of disease. And you will innocently submerge a limb into the miasmic swill to right an upset plastic diver. And then they will have their way.

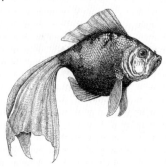

Mycobacteria marinum (mi''-ko-bak-te'-re-ah mar'-i-num), one of several species of mycobacteria that cause *mycobacteriosis* (mi''-ko-bak-te''-re-o'-sis), primarily afflicts fish, causing swelling in their organs, scale loss, emaciation, spinal disfigurement, and eventually death. However, the bacteria do not discriminate, and your fish know this. If they come in contact with an open cut or sore on your arm (or any other extremity), the mycobacteria will invade your body, causing painful boils and pus-filled ulcers in the affected area, and you will have a hell of a time getting rid of your new case of mycobacteriosis. It doesn't respond well to antibiotics, so it often lasts for several years. Even when it is finally eradicated, its effects will linger, in the form of disfiguring scars.

PROGNOSIS

Once the mycobacteria enters your skin, it will incubate for several weeks, multiplying beneath the surface. When it finally emerges, it will resemble a cluster of insect bites—tiny, yet very sensitive, lumps. These will grow into painful open sores, oozing pus. The mycobacteriosis will spread across the affected area and into your joints, causing septic arthritis and deteriorating the underlying bone. In severe cases, it may enter your bloodstream and spread throughout the body, resulting in death.

PREVENTION

Wash your hands thoroughly with bacterial soap after coming in contact with any water or fish that may have been infected. Avoid the stagnant water in which the mycobacteria thrives. Do not get into a hot tub with anybody covered in pus-filled sores.

Mycobacteria marinum are very persistent bacteria. Once they are inside you, they do not want to leave. It will usually take years to get them completely out of your system.

Meanwhile, the affected area should be aspirated—poked with a needle until the pus drains out—and antibiotics such as trimethoprim-sulfamethoxazole and Biaxin 500 should be taken orally. If these fail to remove the mycobacteria, all affected areas may need to be cut out surgically.

After a full recovery is achieved, you will need reconstructive surgery or skin grafting to remove the resulting scars.

Of Note . . .

In the past, outbreaks of mycobacteriosis have been caused by improperly tended swimming pools, but these have been mostly eliminated due to the now common practice of treating pools regularly with chlorine. However, several recent outbreaks have been linked to nail salons. After receiving pedicures, many customers have found their lower legs covered with unsightly disfiguring sores, a result of submerging their feet in the whirlpool baths that precede the pedicures.

NECROTIZING FASCIITIS

(ALSO FLESH-EATING DISEASE, FLESH-EATING BACTERIA)

In which your flesh begins to decay while you're still alive.

SYMPTOMS

- discomfort
- sensitivity
- pain
- discoloration of the skin
- swelling
- blistering
- rash
- fever
- sore throat
- nausea
- vomiting
- diarrhea
- dehydration
- malaise
- weakness
- muscle pain
- decreased urination
- rapid heart rate
- decreased blood pressure

DIAGNOSIS

Yes, putrefaction is a necessary part of your body's decomposition process and is integral to the cycle of life. But, one would think that bacteria would have the good taste to wait until you're dead to begin eating away at your flesh. When bacteria, such as *Group A Streptococcus* (strep''-to-kok'-us), decide, *The hell with waiting for death; I'm going now*, well, that's just tacky.

This is called *necrotizing fasciitis* (nek'-ro-tiz"-ing fas"-e-i'-tis), and it means "decaying infection of the fascia" or "bacteria eating the connective tissue of your flesh while you're still alive to feel it happening." Both definitions are equally correct. The bacteria enters your skin through any size cut or abrasion; it could be something as small as a paper cut or a bruise on your shin from bumping into a chair in the middle of the night. The *Group A Streptococcus* then multiplies quickly. It soon starts to release toxins and enzymes that begin the decaying process beneath your skin and spread to the surface as blisters filled with a dark fluid and warm, discolored gangrenous sores.

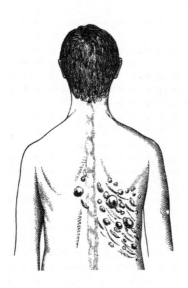

NECROTIZING FASCIITIS

PROGNOSIS

You may very well die. The toxins released by the bacteria could cause your organs to go into systemic shock, resulting in respiratory, renal, and heart failure. But, let's assume that doesn't happen. Okay, good. You still might need to have one or more of your limbs amputated to stop the quick spread of decay.

PREVENTION

There are two effective ways to prevent necrotizing fasciitis. One is to avoid all minor and major cuts and bruises. Since this is just next to impossible to do, you might as well just ignore that suggestion.

The other is to avoid *Group A Streptococcus* bacteria. Since about a quarter of all people are carrying the bacteria at any given time, that's also pretty much impossible, so you can go ahead and ignore that one, too. See, not everybody who carries *Group A Streptococcus* bacteria shows symptoms, but that doesn't mean that you won't get necrotizing fasciitis if they pass it on to you. All they'd have to do is breathe on your newly pierced ear, and the next thing you know, you've got it.

So, really, there are no effective ways to prevent necrotizing fasciitis. All you can do is wash often with an antibacterial soap and keep your fingers crossed (but not so tightly that they bruise).

TREATMENT

Have the infected flesh cut off and thrown away. This will prevent the disease from spreading to other areas. Preferably, this should be handled by a doctor, or at least someone who really thinks he knows what he's doing.

If caught early enough, antibiotics such as penicillin, aminoglycoside, cephalosporin, or metronidazole may hold the damage to an acceptable minimum. The problem is that in its early stages necrotizing fasciitis resembles influenza, so it usually goes unnoticed until it's too late for antibiotics. (Note: If you have the flu, do not begin hacking away at your flesh as a prophylactic measure.)

Of Note . . .

Group A Streptococcus is the exact same bacteria that causes the rather common strep throat and impetigo. Enjoy your day.

THE PLAGUE
(ALSO THE BLACK DEATH)

In which rats and fleas infect you with a very historically significant disease.

SYMPTOMS

- swollen lymph nodes
- fever
- chills
- nausea
- vomiting
- headaches
- body aches
- coughing
- coughing up blood
- weakness
- lethargy
- exhaustion
- black patches on skin

DIAGNOSIS

Remember that bacterial disease that swept through Europe in the Middle Ages? Didn't it kill, like, several million people across the continent before it finally subsided? It was called the Black Death, wasn't it? It's nice to know that the Black Death is gone for good. Just a chapter in your history books. Hey, wouldn't it suck to find out that somewhere between one thousand and three thousand people still die from the Black Death every year? And it would *really* suck to hear that a couple people just died from it in *New York City* in 2002. Thank God *that's* not the case, so everyone can go on living their lives in the peaceful bliss of a Black Death-less existence. Right?

Okay, so it turns out that the Black Death, or the Plague, still does exist. And, yes, it does kill a couple thousand people every year. At least it has very definite symptoms that are easy to recognize and are not all similar to the symptoms of common illnesses like the flu or a cold. And it's really nice to know that the Plague can't kill you on *the very same day* that the symptoms appear. And that there's *no way* that the Plague can become airborne through an infected person's coughs or sneezes. So, there's really nothing to worry about. Sorry, what's that?

Oh.

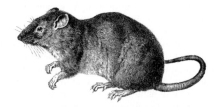

PROGNOSIS

The Plague usually enters the body through the bite of a flea infected with the bacteria *Yersinia pestis* (yer-sin'-e-ah pes'-tis), and commonly begins as bubonic plague (bu-bon'-ic plag), causing fever, chills, and buboes (or swollen, hot-to-the-touch lymph nodes) on the groin, armpit, or neck within about a week. Sometimes the buboes come a few days after the other symptoms, so it's rather easy to confuse the disease with a case of the flu. If this is not dealt with quickly, it will often seep into the bloodstream, causing septicemic plague.

Septicemic plague (sep''-ti-se'mik plag) must be treated immediately because it moves very quickly, wasting no time in turning you into a cadaver, sometimes within a day. Victims of this form often have patches of black skin where blood has seeped into the skin. Septicemic plague does not always follow bubonic plague, and sometimes it precedes it.

When the *Yersinia pestis* bacteria spreads into the lungs, it leads to pneumonic plague (nu-mon'-ic plag), which is very dangerous because in this form, it can be coughed or sneezed into the air on the subway or in a crowded elevator. People who inhale these airborne droplets can become infected with pneumonic plague and then spread it to other people. Symptoms are similar to bubonic plague, but include respiratory problems, such as a severe cough and bloody sputum.

In any of these cases, the bacteria will ravage the body and cause death about a week after the onset of symptoms.

PREVENTION

Try to avoid being bitten by fleas that have recently been fraternizing with rats. The fleas become infected by feeding off the blood of infected rats or other animals, and once the animal dies, the fleas look for another blood host. Also try not to get bitten by an infected rat, dog, or cat. Even handling them or their carcasses may cause infection, so think about that the next time a buboe-covered dog carcass catches your eye. If a person whom you suspect has the Plague coughs, hold your breath and walk out of the room.

TREATMENT

If caught early, the Plague can be handled easily with an antibacterial drug such as streptomycin or gentamicin. After that, forget about it.

Of Note . . .

The Plague has played a major part in history. Besides killing millions of Europeans during the Middle Ages, it is also believed to have been the Hebrew God's punishment for the Philistines for having stolen the Ark of the Covenant. Plague victims were hurled from catapults into cities under siege by medieval armies. And, after World War II, both the United States and the Soviet Union were working on ways to use pneumonic plague as a biological weapon against the other. It is, in fact, still a dangerous and possible threat as a biological weapon.

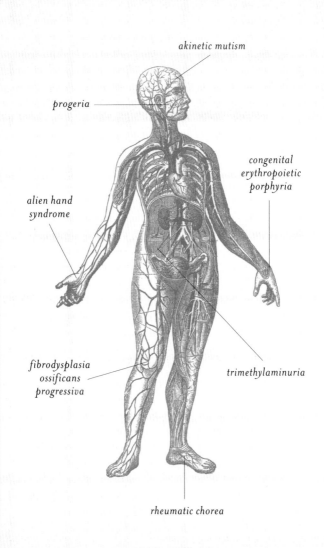

GENETIC & NEUROLOGICAL

In which your body causes its own demise through faulty DNA, a brain defect, or an overachieving immune system.

AKINETIC MUTISM
(ALSO COMA VIGIL)

*In which you spend the rest of your days unspeaking and
wide awake, but unable to move.*

SYMPTOMS

- loss of speech
- incontinence
- loss of motor skills
- weakness

DIAGNOSIS

Akinetic is a medical term referring to an unmoving state,
and *mutism* refers to an unspeaking state. If you put those
two words together, you get a very boring party guest.

Akinetic mutism (ah''-ki-net'-ik mu'-tizm) is a neurological disease in which the victim is unable to talk or move,
though he or she will follow normal sleep patterns. During
the waking hours of the sleep pattern, the victim will, by
all accounts, be awake, but will not move or talk. His or
her eyes will even follow action around the room. It's not a
physical disability, like paralysis. Victims have the physical
ability to stand up and tell everybody to just quit it with all
the medical tests and stuff; they just *don't,* because their brain
won't let them. Though this all may be very frustrating for
the victim's family and friends, and they may swear that the

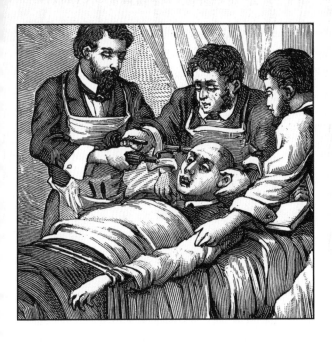

victim is just being terribly stubborn, no amount of shaking or bribing will be able to snap the victim out of it. Not even the original studio soundtrack to *Jesus Christ Superstar*, which is, as anybody who knows anything knows, far superior to the movie soundtrack.

It's not known for certain how cognizant the victim is of everything happening around him or her, because victims tend to be annoyingly obstinate about not answering questions.

PROGNOSIS

Sorry, but if you get this, it's not looking very good for you. You will most likely spend a full and otherwise healthy life bedridden, immobile, and unspeaking. The good news is that you're not really in a coma, so it's quite possible that you'll be wide-awake and fully aware of everything that's happening around you. The bad news is that you're not really in a coma, so it's quite possible that you'll be wide awake and fully aware of everything that's happening around you.

PREVENTION

Keep that brain safe. Akinetic mutism is usually caused by bilateral damage to the orbital surface of the frontal lobes, and nobody wants that. This damage can occur as a result of any number of things, including carbon-monoxide poisoning, drug overdose, Creutzfeldt-Jakob disease (page 182), arboviral encephalitis (page 186), and having your head smashed into a plane of asphalt after being hurled from a motorcycle.

In most cases, akinetic mutism is incurable. However, treatments with levodopa, bromocriptine, or trihexyphenidyl have been known to do some good, but those drugs are pretty hard to score. They're also not very good at getting you in the proper mood while listening to *Jesus Christ Superstar*.

GENETIC & NEUROLOGICAL

"You will most likely spend
a full and otherwise healthy
life bedridden, immobile,
and unspeaking."

ALIEN HAND SYNDROME
(ALSO ANARCHIC HAND)

In which your own hand may attempt to choke you to death.

SYMPTOMS

- impaired judgment
- loss of motor skills
- memory loss
- behavioral changes
- emotional changes

DIAGNOSIS

If you happen to contract *alien hand syndrome,* it may feel as though a demonic spirit has taken control of one of your arms, but don't worry. It's more likely that your brain has been so badly damaged by any one of a number of neurological traumas, such as a stroke or having a green marble cigar ashtray slammed against your skull, that the two halves are not functioning properly; and therefore a dormant personality is controlling the alien hand's actions and attempting to kill your dominant personality. That's all.

Most people with this neurological disease jump to the conclusion that just because one of their hands is beyond their control and seemingly acting with a mind of its own, that the alien hand has malevolent intent. But this isn't always true. An alien hand won't always try to kill you. Sometimes, it will simply unbutton your blouse or pants in public, or knock food out of your mouth, or poke you in the eye, or masturbate you while you're having a conversation.

Of course, the alien hand may try to kill you. That's definitely a possibility.

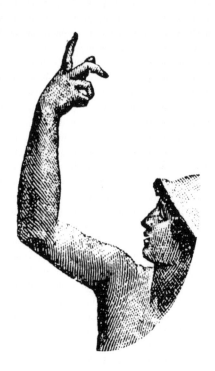

PROGNOSIS

You will not die. Unless the alien hand syndrome is an effect of a brain tumor. In that case, you'll most likely die, but not from the alien hand syndrome; you'll die from the tumor. Or it's possible that your alien hand may grab control of your car's steering wheel and drive you head first into oncoming traffic. It would be pretty easy to imagine you dying in that situation as well. Of course, your alien hand could shove rat poison into your mouth or jam a finger into an electrical socket. Actually, there are lot of things your alien hand can do to make you die, but if it doesn't do any of them, you'll be fine.

PREVENTION

Don't get an infection of the brain or a brain tumor. Don't get brain surgery, particularly not to your corpus callosum, the bundle of nerves that links the left and right sides of your brain. Don't allow any non-water soluble proteins inside your brain (see Creutzfeldt-Jakob disease, page 182). Don't have a green marble cigar ashtray slammed against your skull repeatedly. Don't have a stroke.

There is no treatment for alien hand syndrome. Sometimes it goes away after a few weeks, and other times it lasts for years and years. The only thing that you can do is keep the alien hand occupied. Give it a yo-yo or a stuffed animal to hold.

GENETIC & NEUROLOGICAL

> "Your alien hand could shove rat poison into your mouth or jam a finger into an electrical socket."

Of Note . . .

It has been theorized that the title character in *Dr. Strangelove, or How I Learned to Stop Worrying and Love the Bomb*, played by Peter Sellers, is afflicted with alien hand syndrome, which would explain his involuntary attempts to strangle himself and raise his hand in a Nazi salute.

CONGENITAL ERYTHROPOIETIC PORPHYRIA (ALSO GUNTHER'S DISEASE, CONGENITAL HEMATOPORPHYRIA, ERYTHROPOIETIC UROPORPHYRIA)

In which your skin blisters and burns when exposed to the sun.

SYMPTOMS

- discolored, reddish urine
- discolored, reddish teeth
- sensitivity to sunlight
- blistering
- burning
- rash
- swelling
- abdominal pain
- constipation
- vomiting
- personality changes
- confusion
- hallucinations
- seizures
- numbness
- muscle pain
- weakness
- paralysis

DIAGNOSIS

Congenital erythropoietic porphyria (kon-jen'-i-tal eh-rith"-ro-poi-et'-ik por-fe'-re-ah), a rare disease featuring extreme photosensitivity, is caused by an excess of porphyrins in the blood.

Porphyrins help create much needed hemoglobin and enzymes for the body, but when an excess builds up, your skin burns like hell when exposed to the sun. Sunlight will cause painful blistering, itching, and erosions and may lead to permanent scarring and excessive hair growth. In severe cases, it has caused chronic damage to skin, cartilage, and bone, leading to serious mutilation of the body.

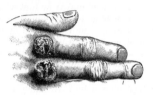

There are seven other types of porphyria, but the congenital erythropoietic type, due to the severity of its effects, is definitely in the upper echelon of those you don't want to get.

This is important: Victims of congenital erythropoietic porphyria are not to be confused with vampires! If one of them doesn't like garlic, that doesn't mean anything; it just means he or she doesn't like garlic. Not everybody likes garlic.

PROGNOSIS

Congenital erythropoietic porphyria will most likely not kill you. However, be very careful to avoid sunlight, as it can lead to severe electrolyte imbalances, low blood pressure, and shock.

CONGENITAL ERYTHROPOIETIC PORPHYRIA CONTINUED

For a victim of this disease, an attack will usually begin with severe abdominal pain, vomiting, and constipation. Personality changes may occur, along with numbness, tingling, weakness, and possibly paralysis. And then there's the whole thing with your skin burning and blistering. Let's not forget that.

PREVENTION

There's no true way to prevent congenital erythropoietic porphyria. It's usually inherited and apparent at birth. However, in some cases, symptoms will not occur until adulthood and may be triggered by alcohol, barbiturates, or a number of other drugs. So, if you're really intent on staying safe, you should consider keeping clean of those drugs.

TREATMENT

First of all, stay the hell away from sunlight. Don't go to the beach. Don't get a job as a roofer. Rethink that vacation to the Grand Canyon. Sunscreens with light-reflective agents may help a bit but won't do the whole job. Wear clothing that covers as much skin as possible. None of this will help cure the disease, but may keep your skin from erupting into painful, disfiguring blisters.

Also, consider covering all your windows with cardboard and duct tape. Go ahead and brick up the windows. Then paint the bricks black. Then cover the black bricks with metal sheeting and paint that black. If you run out of black paint, ask a friend to get more, so you can stay safely inside your darkened home. You can never be too safe.

Porphyria may actually be treated by having bone marrow transplanted to reduce porphyrin production, or by ingesting charcoal to help bind porphyrins in the intestines so they may be excreted more easily.

The paint and bricks are always there as a fallback plan.

Of Note . . .

Camp Sundown is designed specifically for children otherwise unable to enjoy summer camp. The children sleep during the day and engage in activities, such as swimming and horseback riding, from 9 p.m. to 5 a.m. The camp is a project of the Xeroderma Pigmentosum Society in Craryville, New York. Although originally conceived for children with xeroderma pigmentosum, it is available to children suffering from porphyria or any other photosensitivity disease.

FIBRODYSPLASIA OSSIFICANS PROGRESSIVA

In which your muscles turn to bone.

SYMPTOMS

- decreased mobility
- hard lumps beneath skin

DIAGNOSIS

This is the sitting room. The sofa is a genuine Chesterfield, dating back to 1900, fully restored and reupholstered. It was a gift. There, on the wall, is an original Matisse, from his experimental two-dimensional period. And over here is Uncle Walter. What's that? No, it's not a waxwork. It's actually Uncle Walter. Unfortunately, he has fibrodysplasia ossificans progressiva, so most of his muscles have turned to bone, fused to one another. It's some sort of genetic disorder. He can't really do much, so he's usually kept propped up here in the corner. He seems to like it, and he looks rather nice next to the Tiffany stained-glass lamp, don't you think?

Oh, *fibrodysplasia ossificans progressiva* (fi''-bro-dis-pla'-se-ah os'-i-fi-kans pro-gres'-iv-ah) is a disease in which a faulty protein, called BMP, responsible for building and healing bones, mistakenly reacts to any small injury to a muscle or connective tissue. If, say, you were to fall on a patch of ice and sprain your quadriceps, the BMP will react and begin "fixing" the muscle by replacing the damaged area with bone material. You will awaken one morning soon after and find a hard lump protruding from your thigh. Eventually, as more of these injuries occur, these bones will fuse into one another, locking your joints into place, so that you slowly lose mobility.

Not too nice, is it? Now, what do you say to a snifter of Lustau?

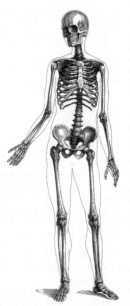

PROGNOSIS

With each small injury to your muscles or connective tissue, a new patch of bone will grow in the damaged tissue's place. Your joints will eventually become fused together. One day, you won't be able to bend your right elbow. The next, perhaps, your left knee. As time goes on, you will lose more and more mobility, until you are permanently locked into place—hopefully, but not necessarily, in a sitting or lying position.

Particularly bad situations may occur if your jaw or throat muscles become affected, as it could make eating, breathing, and living extremely difficult.

PREVENTION

The cause of fibrodysplasia ossificans progressiva is still unknown, but it is believed to be the result of a mutated gene, most likely the one responsible for triggering BMP to build your initial skeleton during child development, but they don't know what is causing it to become active again so much later in life. It just happens. Researchers have eliminated nearly every possible gene that may trigger the disease but still haven't found it. But there are only so many left, so it's got to be coming soon. Until that happens, though, there's still no way to prevent it. Until further notice, you should wear protective padding at all times.

TREATMENT

You might think that you could have surgery to get the new bone tissue separated from your regular skeleton and free up mobility, but any attempt to do so causes BMP to go crazy and start creating bones faster than you can keep up.

However, a protein called noggin (yes, it's called *noggin*), found in the embryos of certain African frogs, has been known to interfere with the process of bone formation, and this has had some helpful effects for victims of fibrodysplasia ossificans progressiva. This may help slow things down enough to make surgery possible.

Of Note . . .

Fibrodysplasia ossificans progressiva is the only disorder known to cause one type of body tissue to change into another type. So, at least you know you're anything but ordinary. For whatever that's worth.

PROGERIA (ALSO WERNER SYNDROME)

In which you look thirty or forty years older than you actually are.

SYMPTOMS

- wrinkling
- withered muscles
- weight loss
- thin skin
- gray hair
- hair loss
- high-pitched voice
- short stature
- cataracts

- excessive thirst
- excessive hunger
- loss of eyesight
- decreased blood circulation
- cold limbs
- fatigue
- premature menopause
- premature aging

DIAGNOSIS

If you are a very lucky person, you will live to see yourself as a very old man or woman. If you are a very *unlucky* person, you will live to see yourself as a very old man or woman, but you'll still be in your thirties or forties.

Progeria (pro-je'-re-ah) typically presents itself in the late twenties or early thirties. Up until that point, you may lead an absolutely normal life, staying up until ungodly hours doing God knows what and not appreciating all the sacrifices your parents made on your behalf. And then you will find that you're aging. Incredibly rapidly.

Your skin becomes wrinkled and pale. You lose your eyesight. Your hair goes gray and begins to collect in the sink. You lose muscle mass and walk stooped over. Your taste in music degenerates, and you find yourself talking to the television as though it's going to answer you. You cannot for the life of you figure out how to use a cell phone, let alone email. What is this email anyway? Can't anybody use a telephone anymore?

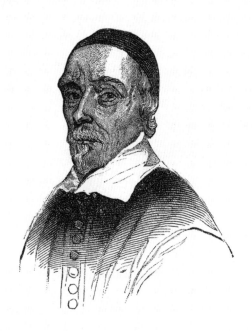

PROGNOSIS

Aging, and its accompanying degenerative effects, will occur rapidly. By the time you're thirty, you'll appear sixty. By the time you're forty, you'll appear eighty. By the time you're fifty . . . well, you probably won't become fifty. Victims of progeria usually die sometime in their late forties.

PREVENTION

There is no way to prevent progeria. It's a genetic disorder. Medical science has not yet proven that it is God punishing you for forgetting your mother's birthday three years in a row. But what do those medical scientists know? Did they carry you in their womb for nine months?

There is no cure for progeria. Individual symptoms may be treated in much the same way that symptoms of aging may be treated. By complaining, mostly.

"Your taste in music degenerates, and you find yourself talking to the television as though it's going to answer you."

Of Note . . .

The upside of having progeria is that you get to take advantage of the senior-citizen discounts at movie theaters and restaurants. Use it while you can.

RHEUMATIC CHOREA
(ALSO SYDENHAM'S CHOREA, CHOREA MINOR, ST. VITUS' DANCE)

In which you lose control of your own body's movements.

SYMPTOMS

- clumsiness
- erratic, uncontrollable movement
- grimacing
- sore throat
- swollen lymph nodes
- fever
- headache
- nausea
- vomiting

DIAGNOSIS

Have you ever had a faulty mouse for your computer? You know that you're *trying* to click on the folder where you keep all your porn, but the cursor never quite makes it there. It jerks erratically around the screen, and you accidentally end up opening the folder containing that novel you never got around to finishing. That's what rheumatic chorea is like, except that instead of the cursor being uncontrollable, it's your body, and instead of the mouse being faulty, it's your brain.

Rheumatic chorea (roo-mat'-ik ko-re'-ah) is a disease of the central nervous system brought upon by *Group A Streptoccocus* bacteria, which also causes necrotizing fasciitis (see page 60). The bacteria infects the body, usually starting as the relatively common strep throat or tonsillitis, but eventually spreads into the spinal cord and brain, where it impedes the brain's ability to control your body's movements. You may have an incredibly difficult time simply lifting a coffee cup to your lips, or buttoning your shirt, or typing your PIN into an ATM machine, which will make everyone waiting in line behind you very annoyed, but not as annoyed as they'll be at the strange convulsive movements you'll make. And you won't be able to help it. Your hands and feet will just be flying everywhere.

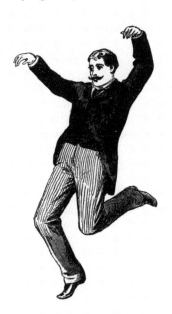

RHEUMATIC CHOREA

PROGNOSIS

It may begin as a simple sore throat, like most people get every winter, but it won't go away. You'll try to pick up your car keys but accidentally knock them to the floor. For no apparent reason, the newspaper will fly from your hands, and when you go to pick it up, you'll knock over your glass of port and kick the dog in the face. People will say, "Why are you grimacing at me?" and you'll say, "I'm not grimacing at you," and they'll say, "Yes, you are." Eventually, it will progress to the point where you can't walk, you can't work, and you can't paint Civil War figurines. Your fingers will be cocked at odd angles and your hands will jerk randomly in front of you, and you'll be completely aware of what's happening but incapable of stopping it. If it gets really bad, you may have to be restrained for your own safety and the safety of others.

PREVENTION

The only way to prevent rheumatic chorea is to prevent yourself from getting a streptococcal infection. This is difficult because so many people carry the streptococcus bacteria, and most of them don't even know it. Somebody could sneeze near you and cause an infection. What you can do is wash yourself regularly with antibacterial soap and have any illnesses that *might* be streptococcal treated early, before they can spread to your brain.

TREATMENT

GENETIC & NEUROLOGICAL

Rheumatic chorea will go away on its own, a few months after the streptococcal infection is treated with antibiotics (such as penicillin or erythromycin). In the meantime, don't play darts, don't carve the Thanksgiving turkey, and don't carry vials of sulfuric acid from one end of the laboratory to the other.

Of Note . . .

The word *chorea* is Greek for "dancing." The disease was originally thought to be related to dancing manias that swept through Europe from the thirteenth to seventeenth centuries. Victims engaged in frenzied dances through the streets, yelling, cursing, and making obscene gestures for several days. They would often end their dancing in front of chapels dedicated to St. Vitus, and thus the syndrome received the name St. Vitus' dance. There is little evidence to show that the old St. Vitus' dance is related to the new St. Vitus' dance.

TRIMETHYLAMINURIA

(ALSO FISH ODOR SYNDROME, FISH MALODOR SYNDROME, STALE FISH SYNDROME)

In which your body produces a pungent fishy odor.

SYMPTOMS

- a fishy odor
- annoyed glares from coworkers

DIAGNOSIS

If you wake up and your bedroom smells like fish, and then you take a shower and your bathroom smells like fish, and then you drive to work and your car smells like fish, and then sit at your desk and your office smells like fish, there are two possible explanations: 1) You are being stalked by an angry tuna; or 2) *You* smell like fish. If the latter is the case, it's very likely that you have trimethylaminuria.

Trimethylaminuria (tri''-meth-il-am'-in-ur'-e-ah) is a metabolic disorder in which your body lacks the enzyme responsible for breaking down trimethylamine, the compound that gives fish their familiar odor. Your body produces trimethylamine while metabolizing choline (typically found in foods such as eggs, liver, and soybeans) and trimethylamine-oxide (typically found in fish). If it is not properly broken down by your liver, it will build up in your body and eventually be excreted in your urine, breath, and sweat. Hence, the fishy odor.

For some victims of trimethylaminuria, the effects of the disease wax and wane depending on present circumstances (such as stress levels and diet). For others, the odor is strong and persistent. Trimethylaminuria appears to be more common in women than in men.

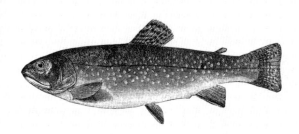

PROGNOSIS

Apart from the smell, there's really not much else to this disease. Granted, it's hard to discount the smell. But if you can, the disease isn't really that bad.

There is a possibility that the disease has other, hidden symptoms. Although trimethylaminuria is a very old disease, dating back at least several centuries, it has only been during the last few decades that it has been taken seriously by the medical community, so it's still being researched. There is some suspicion that the missing enzyme in question (flavin-containing monooxygenase 3) is also needed to break down substances such as antidepressants and nicotine, which could mean that a victim of trimethylaminuria could, when using those substances, experience their common side effects (such as nausea, dizziness, and loss of sexual appetite) to an exaggerated degree or experience side effects that are completely unexpected.

PREVENTION

Trimethylaminuria is caused by an inherited faulty gene or genetic mutation. In either case, there's no way to prevent it. However, it is possible that it may be acquired due to liver or kidney disease or large doses of the bodybuilding drug L-carnitine. So, keep your liver and kidneys healthy, and don't freebase L-carnitine.

Trimethylaminuria cannot be cured, but its foul-smelling effects can be staved off through careful dietary monitoring. Foods that produce trimethylamine should be avoided or eaten in small quantities. These include liver, eggs, soybeans, whole-grain wheat, and marine fish. Research to this point has found no problem inherent in a steady diet of pork chops and Zagnut candy bars.

Low doses of antibiotics, along with stringent hygiene with a moderate pH-level soap, may also help.

Of Note . . .

For some reason that has not yet been identified by science, people with particularly bad cases of trimethylaminuria have a hard time maintaining romantic relationships.

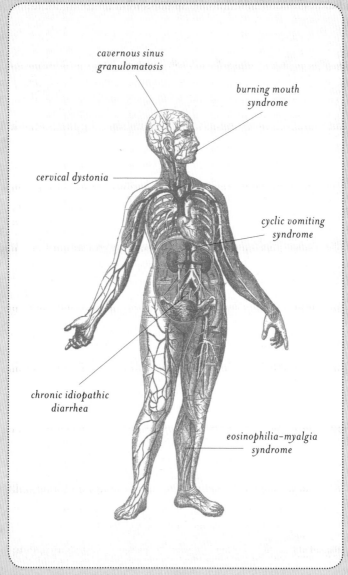

IDIOPATHIC

In which nobody knows why
the hell you're sick, you just are.

BURNING MOUTH SYNDROME

*In which you have a constant painful sensation in your mouth
that lasts for many, many years.*

SYMPTOMS

- dry mouth
- sore mouth
- numb mouth
- altered tastes
- a bitter or metallic taste
- anxiety
- depression

DIAGNOSIS

To date, the only consensus that the medical community has reached about *burning mouth syndrome* is that it freakin' hurts. It is a constant burning sensation in the mouth—on the tongue, the palate, the lips—accompanied by a loss of taste or a bitter, metallic taste.

Imagine rinsing your mouth out with extra-strength bleach. That's how it feels all the time. Or at least most of the time. There's a brief period after you've woken up in the morning when you feel perfectly fine. Almost well enough to believe that the unpleasant ordeal has passed. However, you'll quickly remember from the previous day, or last week, or last month, or last year, that this pain-free

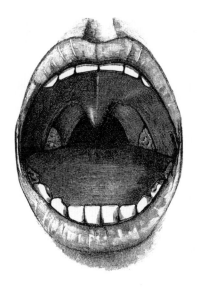

time is deceiving. By mid- to late morning, it will begin to creep back, a familiar slow burn that gains intensity over the course of the day and reaches its height when you most want it to be gone: at night, when you want to sleep. Unfortunately, it won't go away until after you've fallen asleep, and you can't sleep as long as the pain persists. This cycle will occur every day for many years.

BURNING MOUTH SYNDROME CONTINUED

PROGNOSIS

You will live a long and otherwise healthy life full of constant oral pain.

People with the disease have often, and unsurprisingly, reported associated depression, anxiety, irritability, and mood changes.

PREVENTION

Any of the following measures will prove equally effective in preventing burning mouth syndrome: shamrocks, horseshoes, knocking on wood, wishing very hard. The problem is that since its origin is unknown, figuring out how to prevent it is just about impossible.

Some doctors have tried to link burning mouth sensation to a lack of estrogen, zinc, or vitamin C. Others have claimed it is a form of nerve damage, because its onset has been known to follow dental surgery or recent illness. Most doctors, though, are just happy they don't have it.

Since there's no known cure for burning mouth syndrome, you would be better off finding ways to deal with the discomfort than the disease itself. Painkillers have had some positive effects for patients. Other medications that react directly with the nerves of the mouth, such as amitriptyline, clonazepam, and chlordiazepoxide, have had some good results, but no one knows quite why.

In about 50 percent of cases of burning mouth syndrome, the pain will go away on its own after several years. However, in the other half. . .

Of Note . . .

Though it seems counterintuitive, eating may actually offer some temporary relief from burning mouth syndrome. This gives some credence to the guess that the pain may be linked to nerve damage. According to that theory, if a nerve that senses taste were damaged, in the absence of a taste sensation to pass on to the brain, it would send along a pain sensation instead.

CAVERNOUS SINUS GRANULOMATOSIS
(ALSO OPHTHALMOPLEGIA DOLOROSA, TOLOSA-HUNT SYNDROME)

*In which it constantly feels as though someone were driving
a nail into your eyeball.*

SYMPTOMS

- stabbing eye pain
- protruding eyeballs
- headaches
- fever
- nausea
- vomiting
- dizziness
- vertigo
- fatigue
- tingling sensation in forehead
- numbness in forehead
- drooping eyelids
- blurred vision
- double vision
- blindness

DIAGNOSIS

As the saying goes, having *cavernous sinus granulomatosis* (kav'-er-nus si'-nus gran''-u-lo''-mah-to'-sis) is better than being poked in the eye with a sharp stick, but only in that you are not *actually* being poked in the eye with a sharp stick. It's just a remarkably similar sensation. However, one could probably make a decent case that being poked in the eye with a sharp stick is *better* than having cavernous sinus granulomatosis.

The logic would be that whoever was poking you in the eye with a sharp stick would eventually grow bored of poking you and wander off to watch television or something. But with cavernous sinus granulomatosis, the poking will last for days—or sometimes weeks—and it never gets tired of making you feel like someone is poking you in the eye with a sharp stick. It's a constant stabbing pain in your eye, and, no matter what you do, you can't make it stop. So, actually, yeah, that's probably worse.

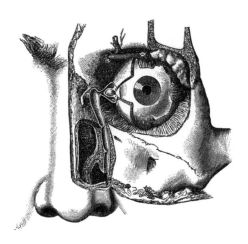

It's caused by an inflammation of the channels that lie behind the eyes: the cavernous sinus and the superior orbital fissure. These channels contain a great number of nerves, so when they get inflamed, the nerves start sending all kinds of crazy pain signals.

PROGNOSIS

First of all, there's the constant stabbing pain to deal with, and that may last for a few weeks. The stabbing pain will usually present itself in only one of your eyes, but if you really luck out it may occur in both.

You should also expect a tingling or numb sensation in your forehead as the cranial nerves respond to the inflammation. Your eyesight may be affected, resulting in blurred or double vision. You may experience permanent cranial-nerve damage, which could lead to long-term vision problems.

PREVENTION

Jeez, that's a tough one. You want to know how you can prevent cavernous sinus granulomatosis? You're on your own here. Doctors know that the inflammation causes the cavernous sinus and superior-orbital-fissure inflammation causes the pain, but they don't know what causes the inflammation. Better luck next time.

Cavernous sinus granulomatosis will usually go away on its own after a few weeks. But, in half the cases, it will come back in a year or so. Corticosteroids taken orally will usually make the effects wane in about two days' time. But, in half the cases, they will come back in a year or so.

In any case, the vision problems and forehead numbness will last a few months. In some cases, they may last forever.

IDIOPATHIC

> "Stabbing pain will usually present itself in only one of your eyes, but if you really luck out it may occur in both."

Of Note . . .

If you suspect that you have cavernous sinus granulomatosis, you should probably get an MRI of your head. It may turn out that all your worrying was for nothing and that instead of inflamed cavernous sinuses and superior orbital fissures, you simply have a brain tumor. Whew. Dodged that bullet, huh?

CERVICAL DYSTONIA
(ALSO SPASMODIC TORTICOLLIS)

*In which your muscles cramp up and twist you into awkward
and painful positions.*

SYMPTOMS

- neck pain
- head shaking
- abnormal posture
- tilted head
- twisted neck

- facial contortions
- loss of motion range
- spasms
- contractions
- pain

DIAGNOSIS

If you think of *cervical dystonia* (ser'-vi-kal dis-to'-ne-ah) as an
extreme case of writer's cramp that, instead of causing your
hand to cramp up while writing letters, manifests itself as severe muscle spasms of your neck, face, and upper chest pulling
your head and shoulders into abnormal, painful positions and
twisting your facial features into a grimace, then it's really not
so bad. If anybody asks you why you look so bizarre, with your
shoulder hunched up high and head twisted to the side at an
angle, you can just tell them you have writer's cramp of the body,
and everyone will have a good laugh (except for you, because
laughing is too painful and may lead to more contractions).

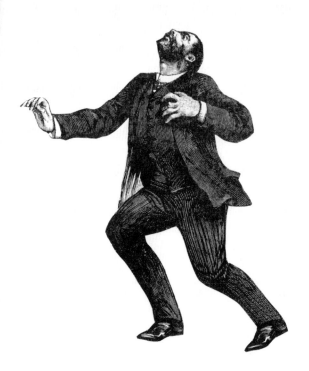

PROGNOSIS

Symptoms of cervical dystonia will come on slowly over the course of months or years; prolonged muscle contractions lasting for minutes or days will pull your body into awkward positions against your will. At first, you may not notice that you're viewing your computer screen from a slight angle or that you're turning to one side to look at your boss straight on. As the disease progresses, it will become more apparent that something is wrong. The spasms and contractions will last longer, grow more painful, and become more pronounced.

Spasms will come and go, usually brought on by specific movements or stress, but almost certainly vanishing completely just before your doctor appointments, leaving you to try to explain your situation to a nodding but unconvinced physician. Eventually, the contractions may become permanent, leaving you twisted into place.

PREVENTION

The exact cause of cervical dystonia is unknown, but it has been hypothesized that it occurs because of abnormal functioning of the brain's basal ganglia. However, why the basal ganglia would do this remains a mystery; they used to be such nice cerebral nuclei.

Cervical dystonia can also, in some cases, be caused by trauma to the brain, such as falling out of a moving roller coaster and landing on your head. For such reasons, you should avoid roller coasters.

There's no real cure for cervical dystonia, but injections of Botox® directly into your muscles may calm muscle activity enough to reduce the spasms. If that doesn't work, surgery may be necessary to intentionally damage parts of the brain that are responsible for the muscle movements.

It's possible that after a few years, your muscles may relax on their own without further spasms, making it seem as though the cervical dystonia has gone into permanent remission. In most cases, though, it will eventually come back.

IDIOPATHIC

Of Note . . .

Botox® is not only a therapeutic medication for cervical dystonia; it's also a cosmetic drug useful for removing unwanted wrinkles and a form of the highly dangerous botulism toxin. The disease Botulism Classic®, useful as an instrument of biological warfare, attacks the nervous system and causes paralysis, which, in turn, leads to asphyxiation and death.

CHRONIC IDIOPATHIC DIARRHEA (ALSO BRAINERD DIARRHEA)

In which you have explosive diarrhea twenty-five times a day.

SYMPTOMS

- diarrhea
- incontinence
- gas
- abdominal pain
- abdominal cramps
- fatigue
- nausea
- vomiting
- fever
- weight loss

DIAGNOSIS

Imagine the worst case of violent, watery diarrhea you've ever experienced. Now, imagine experiencing that worst-diarrhea-ever up to twenty-five times a day. Doesn't sound fun, does it? But wait, because it gets less fun. Now, imagine that worst-diarrhea-ever-twenty-five-times-a-day every day for the next four weeks and having those monthlong episodes occur several times a year for the next two to three years. That's exactly what victims of *chronic idiopathic diarrhea* (kron'-ik id''-e-o-path'-ik di''-ah-re'-ah) have to deal with.

Should you get this disease, take an extended sabbatical from work, cancel your salsa lessons, reschedule your cross-country road trip for about three years from now, and expect to spend many long days within a short jog of a nearby toilet, because you're not going anywhere.

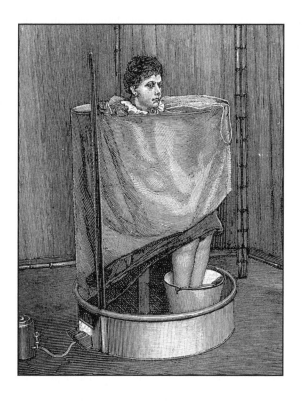

CHRONIC IDIOPATHIC DIARRHEA CONTINUED

PROGNOSIS

You will crap a whole lot. This will be accompanied by massive toilet-paper consumption and a lot of chafing. You'll probably also experience some cramping, nausea, fever, and weight loss. (Chronic idiopathic diarrhea is an excellent way to lose those few extra pounds you've been meaning to shed. A little chronic idiopathic diarrhea after the holidays, and by the time the summer rolls around—three years from now—you'll be in ideal shape for a bikini.)

PREVENTION

Since nobody knows exactly what causes chronic idiopathic diarrhea, it's hard to protect yourself from it. However, because it is thought to be caused by an unknown infectious agent, there are a few things that may help: Don't drink unpasteurized milk. Only drink water that has been chlorinated and boiled and left for fifteen minutes under an ultraviolet lamp. Avoid licking subway poles.

The disease will most likely not spread from person to person, but you probably shouldn't lick subway passengers, either, unless they have been chlorinated and boiled and left for fifteen minutes under an ultraviolet lamp.

There is no known cure for chronic idiopathic diarrhea-except to ride it out. The diarrhea will cease on its own without medicine or curative therapy after anywhere between seven and thirty months, after which time your health should be restored to normal. High doses of loperamide, diphenoxylate, or paregoric have helped to curb the symptoms in some patients.

> "Chronic idiopathic diarrhea is an excellent way to lose those few extra pounds you've been meaning to shed."

Of Note . . .

The first and largest outbreak of chronic idiopathic diarrhea occurred in Brainerd, Minnesota, in 1983. More than 120 people were affected within an eight-month period. Brainerd is also well-known as the setting of the 1996 Coen brothers film *Fargo*, in which Steve Buscemi's character is fed into a wood chipper.

CYCLIC VOMITING SYNDROME

In which you puke all the goddamn time.

SYMPTOMS

- nausea
- vomiting
- gagging
- loss of appetite
- lethargy
- exhaustion
- motion sickness

- sensitivity to light
- headache
- fever
- dizziness
- diarrhea
- abdominal pain
- thirst

DIAGNOSIS

You know the feeling well. It's a churning in the stomach and a lightness of the head. You're cold down in your bones and yet dripping with sweat. Your eyes cannot focus on any fixed point. You find your hand reaching for something to keep you steady, keep you from falling over. And then there's that excessive salivation beneath your tongue. And yet you can't swallow. Without excusing yourself, you push your way across the room, into the hallway, toward the bathroom.

You drop to your knees, shove your face into the porcelain bowl, and push forth a stream of half-digested food. After the contents of your stomach have been emptied, your eyes are blurred with tears, you lean back on your arms and look toward the glistening light fixture. Any normal person would feel relief that the worst has past, but you know that's not the case. This is only the beginning.

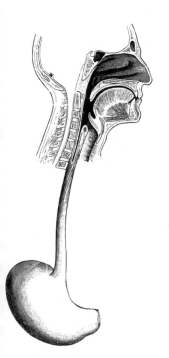

As a victim of *cyclic vomiting syndrome*, you know that the evening out is over. You need to get home, and you may puke a few times on the way. In fact, you'll be puking pretty consistently for the rest of the night, probably through most of tomorrow, and possibly for the rest of the week. You don't know what brought this on—it may have been something you ate or drank, or maybe not—but you know that it's not going anywhere. You'll be spending the next few days either in bed or vomiting, or maybe vomiting in bed. There'll be no work, no jogging, no eating. But, by this point, you're getting used to it.

IDIOPATHIC

PROGNOSIS

About 90 percent of the time, you'll feel absolutely fine. You'll be a completely healthy, active person. However, once you begin to feel that familiar abdominal pain and dizziness, you'll know just what you're heading for. Episodes of excessive vomiting may last for hours or days and will usually weaken your body to the point where nearly any activity—besides puking—is impossible. Eventually, though, it will just go away, and you'll be perfectly functional for several weeks or months. Until the next time.

There may be some long-term effects of the syndrome. For example, the stress of frequent vomiting is likely to cause the lower end of the esophagus to tear open or the stomach to become bruised. And the acids expelled may cause esophageal damage and tooth decay.

PREVENTION

The reasons for cyclic vomiting syndrome are unknown. Nearly anything can trigger an episode, including infection, certain foods, exhaustion, menstruation, and stress. If you can figure out everything that *might* induce an episode, then you should avoid all those things. And good luck with that.

"Eventually, it will just go away, and you'll be perfectly functional for several weeks or months. Until the next time."

TREATMENT

There is no known treatment for cyclic vomiting syndrome. Once you have it, you have it. Individual episodes may be treated. Drugs such as ranitidine and omeprazole, which calm the stomach by reducing acid production, may help. For severe episodes, hospitalization may be necessary, so that you can be monitored and kept hydrated. Propranolol, cyproheptadine, and amitriptyline, which are typically used for migraine sufferers, taken between episodes, may help to curb the syndrome and make episodes less frequent.

Of Note . . .

Diagnosis of cyclic vomiting syndrome is difficult, since it is often confused with other gastrointestinal problems or pledging a fraternity.

EOSINOPHILIA-MYALGIA SYNDROME

*In which severe muscle pains and cramps make it
difficult to play racquetball.*

SYMPTOMS

- muscle pain
- muscle cramps
- joint pain
- itching
- burning sensation
- tingling sensation
- prickling sensation
- numbness
- rash
- coughing

- difficulty breathing
- difficulty swallowing
- indigestion
- diarrhea
- fatigue
- memory loss
- loss of concentration
- hair loss
- hardening of the skin

DIAGNOSIS

You're going to need a very comfortable bed, with lots of
table space around it. Make sure that you can reach things
easily. Have a book handy. A long one. Make certain that your
remote control has fresh batteries, and plan your television
schedule in advance for the next couple of months. (Don't
forget: There's a *Sixteen Candles/Breakfast Club/Pretty in Pink* triple

feature coming up in August!) Settle in and get comfortable. Because you're not going anywhere for a long time.

Eosinophilia-myalgia syndrome (e"-o-sin"-o-fil'-e-ah mi-al'-je-ah) causes severe muscle pain, muscle cramps, skin rash, digestive problems, memory loss, hair loss, and a thickening of the skin (similar to that seen in scleroderma—page 30). This is really a one-stop-shopping answer for symptom collecting. If you're only planning to get one disease this year, get eosinophilia-myalgia syndrome.

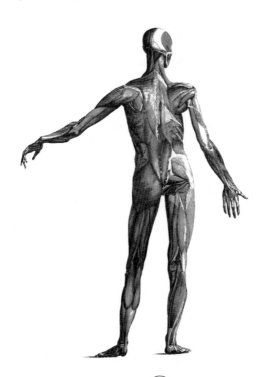

EOSINOPHILIA–
MYALGIA SYNDROME
CONTINUED

PROGNOSIS

The muscle pain and cramps will begin to wane after a few
months, but then they'll flare back up again. You may very
well end up bedridden, unable to do anything physically
productive. And not just because even shifting positions
can cause a spasm, but also because after about a year, your
muscles will grow incredibly weak and you'll become over-
whelmed with a deep and constant fatigue.

Oh, and the nerve damage and pulmonary complications involved may lead to death.

PREVENTION

Sorry, but nobody knows just what causes eosinophilia-
myalgia syndrome. Most of the cases have been linked to
health supplements (used for insomnia, depression, and
premenstrual symptoms) that contain the amino acid L-
tryptophan, but doctors still haven't figured out what it's
doing, if anything. So, perhaps you should avoid them.

> "If you're only planning to get one disease this year, get eosinophilia-myalgia syndrome."

TREATMENT

Most of the effects of eosinophilia-myalgia syndrome are chronic, so they're not going anywhere. But you may want to try to take various medications for the various symptoms, such as muscle relaxers and pain relievers for the muscle pain and cramps.

Of Note . . .

L-tryptophan is found in many common foods, such as chocolate, bananas, peanuts, and turkey. So, if you really want to avoid eosinophilia-myalgia syndrome, maybe instead of your usual turkey sandwich on sourdough with mayonnaise and avocado, you should get roast beef on rye with Dijon mustard and tomatoes (see Ergotoxicosis—page 171). Mmm . . .

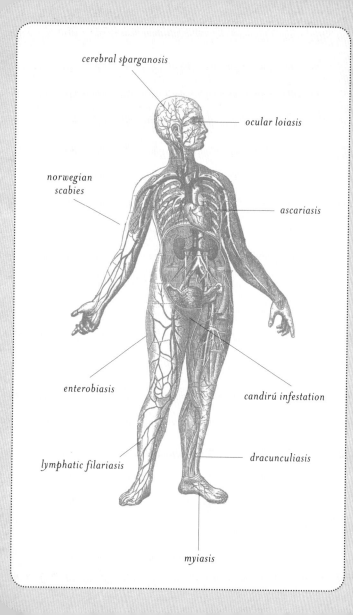

cerebral sparganosis

ocular loiasis

norwegian scabies

ascariasis

enterobiasis

candirú infestation

lymphatic filariasis

dracunculiasis

myiasis

PARASITIC

In which something wriggles and
jiggles and wiggles inside you.

ASCARIASIS (ALSO ASCARIDIASIS)

In which worms climb up from your lungs and through your pharynx in the hopes of being swallowed and laying eggs in your small intestine.

SYMPTOMS

- abdominal pain
- weight loss
- diarrhea
- shortness of breath
- coughing
- fever

- rash
- abdominal cramps
- constipation
- halitosis
- nausea
- vomiting

DIAGNOSIS

Pop Quiz: A female *Ascaris lumbricoides* roundworm is capable of laying two hundred thousand eggs in a single day, and she can do that every day of her adult life, which is approximately one year. Assuming that you have three dozen *Ascaris* roundworms living in you right now, how many eggs will have been produced inside your body by the end of those worms' life spans?[1]

People with *ascariasis* (as''-kah-ri'-ah-sis) have been known to pass large, tangled, wriggling, slimy clumps of the parasitic roundworms from their anus, which can be both satisfying and mind-shatteringly traumatic at once. The *Ascaris*, which grows to eighteen inches in length and resembles the earthworm, spends most of its life in your small intestine, where it mates, lays eggs, and feeds off semi-digested food that passes from your stomach. It will occasionally dig into your intestinal mucous membrane to quench its palate with a little blood.

Most *Ascaris* eggs are excreted with your fecal matter, lying dormant in the soil (or possibly on a toilet seat or door knob) for several years until they are ingested by a new host. Once inside the stomach, they pass into the small intestine,

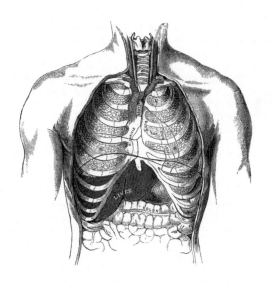

[1] In one year's time, 2,628,000,000 *Ascaris lumbricoides* eggs will have been produced inside you. Of course, this is not counting the eggs of their offspring, or their offspring's offspring.

where they hatch. Larval *Ascarides* will then burrow their way into the circulatory system and eventually the lungs. They cause pulmonary hemorrhaging and respiratory complications as they migrate through the lungs and up the pharynx, in the hopes of being swallowed so that they can re-enter the digestive tract and finally settle for good in the small intestine to live out the rest of their days.

PROGNOSIS

You may very well die, particularly if the larvae cause *pneumonitis* (an infection of the lungs) while migrating through your lungs. At the very least, you will experience gastroenterological problems such as cramps, nausea, and diarrhea. You may also experience some degree of weight loss, as *Ascaris* consumes your food as it passes from the stomach. If enough of the roundworms take up residence in your intestines, it is possible to starve to death even though you're eating regularly.

The worms have also been known to block the intestines' bile and pancreatic ducts, causing peritonitis, a potentially fatal infection of the abdominal membranes. People with intestinal blockage may experience some *copremesis*, also known as vomiting up feces.

PREVENTION

Do not eat food. This is how *Ascaris* eggs enter the digestive system, where your stomach's acids dissolve the eggs' shells and help to hatch the roundworm larvae. Vegetables are especially dangerous, as soil is often fertilized with infected feces.

TREATMENT

There is no universally accepted treatment for ascariasis. Benzimidazoles, mebendazole, and albendazole have been known to help rid *Ascaris* from the intestines, but for *Ascaris* in the lungs, drug treatment can be risky, as decaying larvae may be more dangerous to the body than allowing them to enter the intestines. Chemotherapy has also proven to help clean the body. In severe cases, the roundworms may need to be removed surgically.

Of Note . . .

Ascaris worms are very sensitive to anesthetics. It is not uncommon in surgical recovery rooms to find the roundworms attempting to flee a patient's body through the mouth or nose. At other times, the worms may squirm out into the air and have a look around just for the hell of it.

CANDIRÚ INFESTATION

In which you don't even want to know what happens.

SYMPTOMS

- bleeding
- extreme pain
- terribly extreme pain

DIAGNOSIS

Please, take this advice: skip past this chapter. Turn the page and read the next one on cerebral sparganosis; it's a perfectly horrible disease and will almost certainly satisfy any morbid curiosity you may be harboring. Really, you don't want to know about candirú infestation. You can go the rest of your healthy life without the slightest insight into this terrible malady and will be none the worse for it. So, please, just skip ahead.

Are you still reading? Well, consider yourself duly warned. The *candirú* (kan-dee''-roo), commonly referred to as the vampire fish, is a thin species of catfish that swims up your urethra and lodges itself into your urinary tract. This hurts. A lot. Even if you manage to grab hold of its slippery tail, there's little chance of pulling it out, due to the backward-pointing spines of its gills, which keep it locked firmly in place. Pull all you want; you're just making its job easier. It counts on those spines, along with its sharp grating teeth, to draw the blood from which it makes its meal.

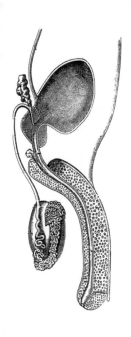

The tiny, eel-shaped, parasitic candirú normally chooses other river fish as its host, squirming between their gills and gorging on their blood, staying there until the fish is dead or candirú has had its fill. It then sinks to the river bottom to rest. It is said, however, that the candirú is attracted to the smell of human urine and that it will follow a stream back to its source, thus finding a human host.

Very little is actually known for certain about the candirú, and different sources have slightly different accounts of its activities and methods. Some accounts have it swimming up the anus instead of the urethra. Others have it swimming against the stream of urine, past the water's surface, to find its unsuspecting host relieving himself on the riverbank.

CANDIRÚ INFESTATION

PROGNOSIS

Expect lots and lots of pain. The candirú will be up inside you, sucking at your blood and flesh, raking its teeth across the mucous membrane of your urinary tract and swelling in size the more it eats. The hemorrhaging that occurs may very well induce death. Even if it doesn't, the pain involved may inspire death.

PREVENTION

Do not pee in the water while swimming, particularly not in the Amazon or Orinoco Rivers in South America, where the fish is most prevalent. On second thought, don't even go in the water. On third thought, stay home and rent a movie. It's much safer.

TREATMENT

Because of the candirú's backward-pointing spines, which it unfurls like an umbrella, you're not going to pull it out. So, forget that. You may also have the fish cut out surgically, but this is a very costly and complicated procedure. One doctor claims to have had to slice into a patient's bladder to remove the fish. Some victims of candirú infestation have simply chosen to have their penises cut off rather than deal with all the unpleasantness.

Another option is a folk remedy used by the people of the Amazon. The fruit of the jagua tree may be brewed into a tea and consumed, so that when you urinate, it causes the candirú to dissolve away inside you. A similar folk remedy is the insertion of the buitach apple into the urinary tract, causing the same dissolving effect. By all accounts, this is very painful and may cause shock and death itself.

Of Note . . .

There are supposedly bans being sought by some people that would make it illegal to import the candirú into the United States. The concern is that some might find their way into U.S. rivers and begin breeding. Because the candirú has no natural enemies and its population could possibly grow unfettered, this would cause quite a problem. Why anybody would want to import these horrible things remains a mystery.

CEREBRAL SPARGANOSIS

In which a parasitic flatworm lives inside your brain.

SYMPTOMS

- headache
- seizures
- cranial pressure
- dementia
- confusion
- decreased intelligence
- speech disturbance
- memory loss

DIAGNOSIS

There are very few instances in which you should count yourself lucky to discover that you have a parasitic flatworm living inside your liver. That said, if you should discover that you have a *Spirometra mansoni* flatworm living inside your liver, get down on your knees and thank God; at least it's not living inside your brain.

The *Spirometra mansoni* flatworm's general aim is to make it into the body of an animal host, such as a dog or cat. However, they will settle for humans if that's what they're presented. The microscopic larvae hang out in bodies of water, after migrating from dog and cat feces, and wait to be ingested by copepods—tiny, shrimp-like crustaceans called water fleas. This is just the beginning of their journey. The copepods are then ingested by an amphibian, such as a frog, or a reptile, bird, or small mammal. The larvae are then passed from animal to animal along the food chain, until they are eaten by their ultimate host, usually a dog or cat, but possibly you, where they can grow to up to fourteen inches in length and a fraction of an inch in width. *Spirometra* can also enter humans directly through contact with infested water or an infected animal.

Once inside your body, the worms will cause some pain as they grow to their adult size and migrate around, looking for a nice place to settle. It's rare for a *Spirometra* flatworm to settle in a human brain, but it has been known to occur.

PROGNOSIS

Cerebral sparganosis (se-re'-bral spar''-gah-no'-sis) can either feel like nothing at all, or it can feel like your intellect is being eaten away from the inside out. It has to do with whether you've got a lazy slacker tapeworm that's content to hang out and chill inside your head or a real go-getter tapeworm looking to make things happen, such as causing seizures, dementia, and random havoc to your intellectual functions as it slithers around in there.

PREVENTION

Boil all water that you drink or bathe in or even touch, especially if it appears to be infested with the microscopic, nearly invisible *Spirometra mansoni* larvae. Avoid contact with dogs and cats that have been outside, especially if they may have had contact with infected water or eaten an infected animal while you weren't watching them. If you are planning to eat any infected animals, such as amphibians, reptiles, birds, or wild mammals, be certain to cook them properly. Refrain from rubbing the flesh of a dead frog into open wounds, regardless of how appealing it may seem.

Cerebral sparganosis is usually treated with surgery; cutting open the skull and manually pulling the flatworm from the brain. There are no known drugs for treating the disease.

> "Refrain from rubbing the flesh of a dead frog into open wounds, regardless of how appealing it may seem."

PARASITIC

Of Note . . .

Non-cerebral sparganosis is sometimes thought to be a tumor, due to the flatworm's shape and texture when coiled, but once the area is cut open and the worm spills out, the confusion usually clears up pretty quickly.

DRACUNCULIASIS
(ALSO GUINEA WORMS DISEASE)

*In which a three-foot-long worm emerges from your ankle
to spew forth its milky white larvae.*

SYMPTOMS

○ fever
○ swelling
○ pain

○ joint pain
○ locked joints

DIAGNOSIS

The problem with *dracunculiasis* (drah-kung''-ku-li'-ah-sis)
is that most people refuse to look on the bright side of the
disease. Sure, you can focus on the crippling pain and the
blistering and the fevers and the millions of tiny larvae that
are spewed into the water every time you take a bath. On the
other hand, you get your own pet worm that goes everywhere
that you go. You can name it (Vladimir, Wormy, etc.). You
can sing songs to it ("I've Got You Under My Skin," "Killing
Me Softly," etc.). And anytime life starts getting you down
(like when you think about the terrible debt you've fallen into
because you're in too much pain to walk, let alone work), you
can just look down at the pus-filled blister on your leg and see
your bestest friend poking its head out, smiling up at you.

The *Dracunculus medinensis* is a parasitic worm that resembles a very long piece of spaghetti. It enters your body in the larval form, hidden away inside fresh-water copepods. When you accidentally ingest the water fleas, your stomach digests the fleas but not the worm larvae. Then the larvae wiggle off to enjoy their new home (you) while growing to adult size, anywhere from two to three feet in length. This takes about a year, during which time the male worms will die after mating. The female worms will migrate to the surface of your skin, usually somewhere on your lower legs, and push their heads out to ejaculate a milky white liquid full of millions of baby *Dracunculus* worms whenever they contact water. The larvae are eaten by water fleas, and then the water fleas are ingested by somebody else, and the whole thing starts all over again.

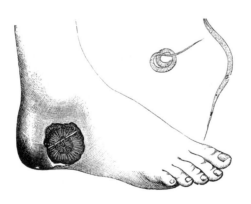

DRACUNCULIASIS

PROGNOSIS

Pain. Expect pain. A three-foot-long worm migrating through your joints does not feel good. Add to that the burning blister that appears on the spot where the worm emerges, which will, more often than not, become infected. These infections complicate matters and bring on other illnesses, some of which could result in death. Or more pain. Usually pain.

Complications from having the worm moving around inside you may also cause permanent crippling.

PREVENTION

Don't drink water infested with water fleas. Don't drink water that you suspect is infested with water fleas. Don't drink water that could maybe be infested with water fleas. Don't drink *with* water fleas (as they are rowdy, unreasonable drunks and may try to jump into your mouth while you're trying to explain that last call was an hour ago).

"Pain. Expect pain."

Unfortunately, your little friend will have to go. The problem is you can't just pull it out at once, because it's so long and thin it will most likely tear in half inside you. Having the calcified remains of your pet worm inside you is even more painful than having a live pet worm inside you. The way to remove the worm is to pull it out bit by bit for several weeks. The traditional method is to wrap the exposed portion of the worm around a small stick and wind it an inch or so every day.

PARASITIC

Of Note . . .

There is some belief that dracunculiasis was, at least in part, the inspiration for the universal symbol for healing, the ancient staff of Asklepios, which portrays one snake wrapped around a stick. Since *dracunculus* is Latin for "little dragon," this could explain the confusion between a three-foot-long worm and a snake.

ENTEROBIASIS (ALSO OXYURIASIS, SEATWORM INFECTION, PINWORM INFECTION)

In which pinworms squirm out of your ass at night to lay their eggs in the folds of your anus.

SYMPTOMS

- itching
- irritability
- restlessness

- abdominal pain
- loss of appetite
- weight loss

DIAGNOSIS

One out of every ten people who pick up this book is currently infected with *Enterobius vermicularis* (en"-ter-o'-be-us ver-mi'-cu-lah"-ris) pinworms. Even if you aren't infected, there's a fifty percent chance that you have been or will be infected at some point in your life. But don't worry. The pinworms probably won't do you much harm. They just want to be left alone to live inside your colon and crawl out of your ass at night to lay their eggs in your anus' warm folds of skin. It's not really much with which to concern yourself.

There is a very simple—beautifully simple, actually—cycle to *enterobiasis* (en"ter-o-bi'-ah-sis). You touch a car-door handle or a glass or a movie-theater armrest, or, yes, even a book, that is infected with *Enterobius vermicularis* eggs. Then, when you put your fingers in your mouth, you allow the eggs to enter into your body, hatch in your small intestine, and migrate to your colon where they mate. The half-inch-long female pinworms climb out into the open air and lay their eggs and then head back inside your ass. Their movement causes irritation and itching, and you (without waking) scratch the itch. Then, when you (also possibly without waking) put your fingers in your mouth again, you re-infect yourself, and the cycle of life continues.

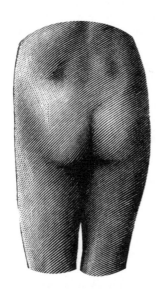

PROGNOSIS

Usually, the worst that enterobiasis gets is some uncomfortable itching, disturbed sleep, and unpleasant-smelling fingers. However, if you get enough pinworms living and mating inside your digestive tract, it could lead to abdominal pain and a loss of appetite.

PREVENTION

Wash your hands immediately after doing anything. Also, refrain from putting your fingers inside the anus of anybody who you think might be infected. If you must, then wash your hands immediately afterward.

The pinworms cannot survive extreme temperatures, so you may want to consider keeping all of your bedding materials in an industrial-quality flash-freezer while not in use.

> "Refrain from putting your fingers inside the anus of anybody who you think might be infected. If you must, then wash your hands immediately afterward."

The best thing to do is bathe, or at least wash your hands, immediately after waking in the morning. Change your underwear daily, and wash your bedclothes and sheets often. Sleep with a cork in your anus. If you can stop the cycle, the worms should die off within a few months.

Anthelmintic drugs, such as mebendazole and pyrantel, have also been effective in killing off the worms.

Of Note . . .

Enterobius vermicularis are so small and light that they can become airborne in a light and fragrant springtime breeze.

LYMPHATIC FILARIASIS
(ALSO BANCROFTIAN FILARIASIS)

In which parasitic worms climb inside your lymph nodes and make your testicles swell to the size of a basketball.

SYMPTOMS

- soreness
- itching
- fever
- chills
- nausea
- vomiting

- diarrhea
- fatigue
- swelling
- incredibly enlarged genitals, breasts, and/or limbs

DIAGNOSIS

Given the option of millions of microscopic roundworm larvae swimming around in your bloodstream, or your scrotum growing so large and heavy it hangs down to your knees, which would you choose? If that seems like a really hard choice, then *lymphatic filariasis* (lim-fat'-ik fil''-ah-ri'-ah-sis) is the disease for you!

Here's how it works: A man with one enormous, misshapen leg limps awkwardly down the street when he gets bit on the arm by a mosquito. It then flies off, satiated for the time being, unaware that it has just ingested hundreds of roundworm microfilariae (microscopic, pre-larval worms) with its blood meal. A week or so later, the mosquito is hungry again. It finds you, and before you can squash it beneath your palm, its proboscis pierces your skin, transferring some of its newly acquired microfilariae into your bloodstream.

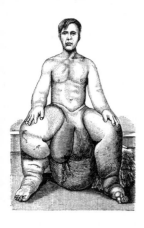

Six months later, completely without your knowledge, the microfilariae have developed into adult *Wuchereria bancrofti* roundworms and have pushed themselves into your lymph nodes, slowly crippling your body's immune system and its ability to regulate a fluid balance between tissues and blood. Two round-worms mate, and the female releases its countless young into your bloodstream.

Months pass; something isn't right. You've been sick all spring—minor illnesses, but illnesses nonetheless—and you are suddenly aware of an exaggerated bulge in your pants. At first, this seems fortuitous. Women flirt with you more regularly. But the bulge continues to grow. It does not stop growing. Your penis and testicles have become unusually large. One might even say *grotesquely large*. They sag heavily beneath your waist. It is now difficult to walk. You limp awkwardly down the street. A mosquito lands on your arm, and you feel its sharp sting. It flies off, satiated for the time being, unaware that it has just ingested hundreds of roundworm microfilariae . . .

PROGNOSIS

Most victims of lymphatic filariasis do not die. So, you've got that going for you. However, the effects of elephantiasis—the condition of having terribly disfigured and enormously oversized limbs or genitals—are not fun. If it's possible for "enormously oversized limbs or genitals" to be considered an understatement, that's exactly what it is. Imagine having testicles the size of an overripe watermelon or a penis that's bigger than your leg.

Besides its unsightly features, elephantiasis can be rather painful. The skin of the affected area will grow hard and thick, discolored and warty. In some cases, the flesh may crack open, leaving you susceptible to any number of bacterial infections, including necrotizing fasciitis (page 60).

On the other hand, it's always possible that having elephantiasis will become fashionable in the near future. All you need is a couple of kids in Brooklyn to sport the disease, and you'll be on the vanguard of style. People will ask you where you got your huge appendage, and you can just shrug off their questions, sip on your Pellegrino, and thank your arthropod benefactor.

It's very easy to prevent lymphatic filariasis. Just don't ever go outside between dusk and dark. That's when the mosquitoes are most active and likely to infect you. That'll get you up to about 99 percent. To ensure that extra one percent of safety, keep your windows sealed shut and wrap yourself in thick rubber sheeting, and then submerge yourself under four feet of water.

TREATMENT

The roundworm parasites can be killed off with the drugs diethylcarbamazine and albendazole. These drugs may also help reduce the effects of elephantiasis, particularly if the disease is treated early. Rigorous cleaning of the affected area may also reduce the effects. How many times do you think you can wash your leg in one day? Thirty-five times? Why not try for thirty-six?

PARASITIC

Of Note . . .

Elephantiasis is sometimes referred to as "wheelbarrow scrotum" due to the fact that many of its victims need wheelbarrows in which to cart around their scrotums.

MYIASIS

In which maggots crawl around beneath your skin.

SYMPTOMS

- pain
- swelling
- sores
- boils

- fever
- itching
- moving sensation beneath the skin

DIAGNOSIS

Some people might say that if you've never experienced the maternal sensation of having a bloated, mature larvae of a flesh fly push its way through your skin, only to fall to the ground and continue its evolution into a fully grown fly—to have nursed a tiny insect into adolescence within your own flesh—you've never really experienced life. Some people *might* say that, but it seems unlikely.

It is a universally accepted truth that maggots are the most disgusting things on earth (narrowly edging out cockroaches and vegan tuna salad). The one place that you really, really don't want maggots is *inside* you, so one disease you definitely don't want is *myiasis* (mi'-yah-sis). This occurs when certain species of flesh flies—such as *Dermatobia hominis* or *Cordylobia anthropophaga*—lay their eggs on your skin, in a body cavity, or directly onto open wounds. The eggs hatch into microscopic larvae and burrow their way beneath the surface and into your body where they do the two things that maggots do best: eat and be creepy.

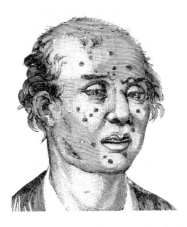

   You might find maggots feeding away under your skin, up your nose, in the gums between your teeth, inside your ear, in your sinuses. That's if you're lucky; maggots have also been found inside the vagina and urethra. In instances of accidental myiasis, when fly larvae are ingested along with infected food, you may find maggots in the intestines or other body cavities. In instances where the fly's eggs were laid directly onto open wounds, they could be anywhere: your foot, your scalp, the side of your face, the tip of your nose.

PROGNOSIS

If you take nothing else away from this book, take this: Having maggots inside of you, eating away at your soft tissue and squirming around a lot in a disgusting manner, is not good for your body. Have you ever seen what maggots do to a dead squirrel on the side of the road? It's itchy, painful, and unsettling. Victims of myiasis have described it as a creeping sensation beneath their skin.

Furthermore, if the maggots make their way up and into your skull, they could cause meningitis, an inflammation of the brain, which could cause death. Or they could simply eat your brain away.

The one positive (read: not incredibly negative) of myiasis is that it's unlikely that you will find fully grown flies swarming out of your nose or ears or vagina. The maggots usually manage to push themselves out of your body before they molt into fully grown flies. Usually.

PREVENTION

People who don't want maggots inside of them are advised to keep all cuts and wounds cleaned and covered. Don't allow any flies to come in contact with exposed wounds. Don't allow flies to land on you, especially not if they look like they want to drop their eggs on your skin. Don't eat food that looks like it may have been infected with microscopic fly larvae. (You may need a microscope to be absolutely certain.)

TREATMENT

The maggots may be forced to leave the body by cutting off their air supply. This may be achieved by spreading Vaseline or oil across the infected area. The maggots will return to the surface to breathe, at which point they may be removed, maggot by maggot, with a pair of tweezers. In particularly bad cases, or when the infestation is internal, surgery may be needed to cut away the infected area.

Of Note . . .

Maggots have been used throughout history for medical purposes. In fact, some doctors still advocate maggot therapy to treat wounds in which the decaying process has already begun. Sterile maggots are packed into the wound and left to eat away the necrotized flesh. The maggots are scooped out and replaced every few days to ensure that they do not develop to maturity inside the body.

Screw that.

NORWEGIAN SCABIES
(ALSO CRUSTED SCABIES)

In which hundreds of thousands of mites burrow their way into your skin.

SYMPTOMS

- pain
- itching
- rash
- sores
- bleeding
- scabbing

- scaling
- flaking
- thickened skin
- disfigured nails
- disturbed sleep

DIAGNOSIS

Some phrases you might find useful during your infestation with *Norwegian scabies* (nor-we'-jen ska'-bez):

Det bor hundretusenvis av små insekter under huden min.
I have hundreds of thousands of tiny insects living beneath the surface of my skin.

Herregud, kløen er ikke til å holde ut! Jeg vet ikke om jeg orker så mye mer.
Sweet Jesus, the itching is unbearable! I don't know if I can take it much longer.

Hold deg unna meg. Jeg
er veldig smittefarlig.
*Please keep your distance. I am
highly contagious.*

Ikke ta på noe i rommet, med
mindre du har lyst til å bli
smittet.
*Don't touch anything in the room,
unless you would also like to become
infected.*

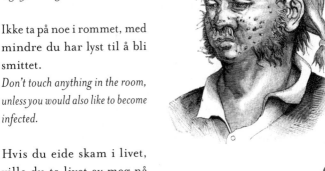

Hvis du eide skam i livet,
ville du ta livet av meg nå
og brenne liket med en flammekaster.
*If you had any decency, you would kill me now and then burn my
corpse with a flamethrower.*

PROGNOSIS

The *Sarcoptes scabiei* (sahr-kop'-tez ska-be'-i) mite—a microscopic eight-legged arthropod that causes normal scabies— is
no different from those that cause the more severe form,
Norwegian scabies. In normal cases you might expect to have

one to two dozen mites living beneath the surface of your skin, usually between your fingers and toes and along your beltline. However, in cases of Norwegian scabies, the mites can number in the hundreds of thousands (or even millions) and be found across the entirety of your body.

As the mites burrow deep into your skin, biting their way through your flesh, leaving eggs and feces behind them as they dig, this can be somewhat uncomfortable. When multiplied a couple hundred thousand times, it sucks as bad as you'd guess it would. Prepare yourself for a lot of itching and some seriously severe allergic rashes.

Your skin will grow calloused and thick, somewhat deformed by your body's hyperkeratotic defense against these insects, particularly on your hands and feet, where your nails will become misshapen and gnarled. Scales of dead skin will fall from your body like snow, making anything you touch infectious to others.

Fortunately (or unfortunately), you won't die.

PREVENTION

Don't go anywhere near anybody you suspect of having Norwegian scabies. Whereas normal scabies is relatively non-contagious, there are so many mites falling from the body of a victim of Norwegian scabies (several thousand a day) that it is extremely contagious. And the mites can live without a human host for several days. So don't touch anything that they touched.

TREATMENT

Because the skin becomes so thick and crusted during infestation, it's difficult to get scabicides (such as benzyl benzoate, permethrin, and aqueous malathion) to penetrate down to kill the mites. You may need to brush or scrape the scales from your skin before applying the lotion.

Of Note . . .

Mennesker har vært plaget av skabbmidd i over 2500 år, og arkeologer har funnet egyptiske tegninger av smittede personer. Det er vidt anerkjent at det var den italienske skipslegen Giovan Cosimo Bonomo som oppdaget årsaken til sykdommen, ut fra tegninger av skabbmidd han lagde i 1687. Man trodde lenge at norsk skabb, eller skorpeskabb, var en type spedalskhet (side 52), siden sykdommen ble observert av den norske hudlegen Daniel Cornelius Danielssen og hans onkel, professor Carl Wilhelm Boeck, i 1848 i en leir for spedalske.

OCULAR LOIASIS
(ALSO AFRICAN EYE WORM)

In which worms live on your eyeball.

SYMPTOMS

- swelling
- discomfort
- itching
- pain
- visual obstruction

DIAGNOSIS

Hey, what's that in your eye? Hold still. It looks like it might just be a piece of lint or something. Wait. There's another one. Hmmm . . . You have a couple of pieces of lint in there. But, if that's lint, why is it wriggling around like that? Oh . . . It's not lint after all. It appears to be a small worm. Or worms, actually. Yes, you definitely have some worms living on your eyeball. Loa Loa worms, to be precise. Perhaps you should be leaving now.

If you're ever on the receiving end of the preceding paragraph, that's too bad for you, because what you have is *ocular loiasis* (ok'-u-lar lo-i'-ah-sis), in which Loa Loa round-worms, or African eye worms, writhe around on or beneath the mucous membrane of your eyeball. This can be very uncomfortable, rather painful, and incredibly creepy. The worm may even migrate its way *through* your eyeball.

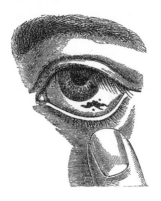

The disease is spread by the deer fly (also known as the mango fly). The female Lao Lao microfilariae circulate through the bloodstream of an infected person, and when the deer fly bites such a person, the fly becomes infected. Then it flies off, and a week or so later, after the microfilariae have molted into larvae, it is ready to infect more people. The larvae enter your body through the deer fly's proboscis and grow to maturity over the course of several years inside your body, usually migrating to your eye, possibly so that they can watch television with you. The more pretentious Loa Loa, the ones that claim not to like television, may migrate to other parts of the body and entertain themselves by causing problems like arthritis, bowel obstruction, or, if they get into the brain, encephalitis (page 186).

PROGNOSIS

The Loa Loa worms can grow to more than two inches in length, so you can imagine how that would feel in your eye. You might find them on the surface of your eye or beneath the surface of your conjunctiva, the clear mucous membrane that covers the inside of your eyelid and the front surface of your eyeball. Besides the physical irritation and visual obstructions involved, the worms may also cause severe facial swelling around the eye that even the best makeup artist would be hard-pressed to hide. Furthermore, the microfilariae may cause ocular inflammation, cataracts, and glaucoma.

PREVENTION

The best way to prevent ocular loiasis is to prevent deer flies from biting you. If you see a deer fly that looks hungry, walk away.

The drug diethylcarbamazine may also be used to prevent infection.

Diethylcarbamazine has been shown to kill both adult Loa Loa worms and their microfilariae. However, this can be dangerous, as it works so quickly that dead microfilariae in your brain can cause capillary blockage, so you die the death of a thousand baby worms in your brain. Ivermectin will also kill the microfilariae, but it doesn't work as fast, so there's less risk of capillary blockage. Albendazole will not only kill the microfilariae, but it will cause the adult Loa Loa to reproduce more slowly.

Alternately, you may have the adult Loa Loa surgically extracted from your eye. A surgeon slices a small slit in your conjunctiva and then pulls the worm out with a pair of tweezers.

PARASITIC

Of Note . . .

The Loa Loa worm was first described in detail by Roger Argyll-Robertson in 1895 after he removed an adult of each sex from the eye of a patient. Because this occurred in Old Calabar, Nigeria, the swellings associated with loiasis are referred to as Calabar swellings to this day.

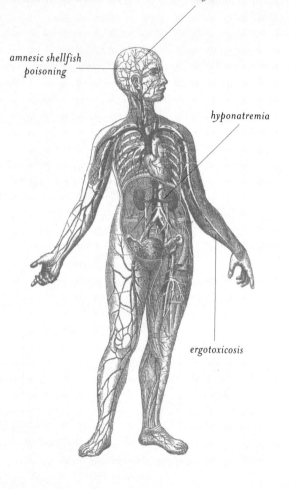

mucormycosis

amnesic shellfish
poisoning

hyponatremia

ergotoxicosis

TOXIC & FUNGAL

*In which a fungus or poison
makes you hate life.*

AMNESIC SHELLFISH POISONING

(ALSO DOMOIC ACID POISONING)

In which you eat some bad scallops and then forget you had anything to eat at all.

SYMPTOMS

- nausea
- vomiting
- abdominal cramps
- diarrhea
- confusion
- dizziness
- disorientation
- weakness
- headaches
- seizures
- memory loss
- dementia
- coma

DIAGNOSIS

You're eating grilled scallops in your favorite seafood restaurant. Or maybe they're steamed clams dripping with melted butter. Or mussels in a spicy tomato sauce, the kind into which you just can't help dipping giant slices of Italian bread. It doesn't really matter. It can be any kind of molluscon filter-feeding shellfish. Anyway, you're enjoying your dinner, and you have no idea that your life, as you know it, is over, thanks to *amnesic shellfish poisoning*.

What you don't realize is that the shellfish you're enjoying

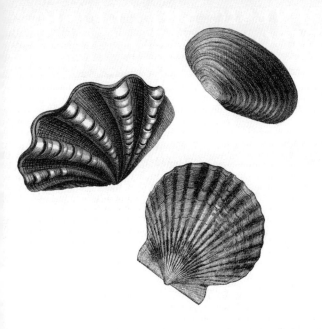

so much with your white wine is filled with domoic acid, a naturally occurring biotoxin found in certain species of algae. The shellfish had sucked in the algae as food, digested it, and kept its toxin stored inside. Then it was caught, shipped to your favorite restaurant, and prepared into the delicious meal you're now eating. The domoic acid poison is already seeping into your own digestive tract, where it will cause nausea and cramping. If you were lucky, that's where it would end. You're not lucky. It will soon move into your nervous system and the brain, attacking the hippocampus directly, compromising its ability to form new memories and process spatial relations.

AMNESIC SHELLFISH POISONING CONTINUED

PROGNOSIS

You should begin to feel the toxins' gastroenterological effects within the first six hours after consumption. You will mostly experience repeated vomiting, but it will feel like it's only happening once. Within a few hours, you'll begin to realize that you can't remember where you left your keys or what you did five minutes ago. Then you'll realize it again. You'll discover that you've lost the ability to learn anything new. Actually, you won't discover that. You won't be discovering anything anymore.

PREVENTION

The only way to truly safeguard yourself from amnesic shellfish poisoning is to not eat shellfish. Not clams, mussels, scallops, or crabs. No amount of cooking or cleaning will neutralize the domoic acid toxin in an infected shellfish.

Infected shellfish look and taste just like regular shellfish. Perhaps a real shellfish aficionado might notice a slight rise in the domoic acidity, but the warnings of people who claim to be shellfish aficionados are seldom paid much attention.

There is no known antidote for amnesic shellfish poisoning.

"Perhaps a real shellfish aficionado might notice a slight rise in the domoic acidity, but the warnings of people who claim to be shellfish aficionados are seldom paid much attention."

Of Note . . .

Recipe for Amnesic Shellfish Poisoning with Garlic and Rosemary: Wash infected shellfish and pat dry. Roll infected shellfish in a shallow bowl of flour. Heat four tablespoons of salted butter over a low flame and add infected shellfish. Let cook for two minutes and begin stirring in minced garlic and rosemary. Cook for another two minutes. Garnish with lemon wedges. Will infect three to four people.

ERGOTOXICOSIS
(ALSO ERGOTISM, ERGOT POISONING, ST. ANTHONY'S FIRE, HOLY FIRE)

In which your limbs feel as though they are on fire and then eventually fall off.

SYMPTOMS

- itching
- burning sensation
- tingling sensation
- prickling sensation
- muscle cramps
- muscle pain
- numbness
- swelling
- diarrhea
- nausea
- vomiting
- headache
- twitching
- convulsions
- vertigo
- depression
- fatigue
- drowsiness
- seizures
- disorientation
- hallucinations
- skin peeling
- skin discoloration
- gangrene
- loss of digits or limbs
- crazy dancing and screaming

DIAGNOSIS

If you've ever shoved your arms into a cauldron of fire while tripping your face off on acid, you might have some idea of what ergotoxicosis (er"-go-tok"-si-ko-sis) feels like. In fact, it's really pretty much the same thing. Should you find yourself poisoned by the fungus *Claviceps purpurea* (klav'-i-seps pur-pur'-e-ah), or ergots, it will affect your body in two ways.

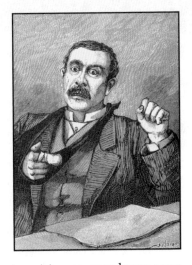

Two toxic alkaloids in the fungus, ergotamine and ertolaline, cause the muscles to constrict, which cuts off the blood supply to your extremities, so your lower arms and lower legs begin to die off while still attached to your body. At the same time, the lysergic acid amide in the fungus affects your brain. Since lysergic acid amide is a very close relative to lysergic acid diethylamide (more commonly known by its acronym, LSD), you are in for some interesting times. If you've never "gone sheet rocking" (common street terminology for using LSD), here's something you should know: extreme hallucinations + severe pain = no fun at all. Victims of ergotoxicosis go goddamn crazy. There have been reports of people running wildly through the streets, crazily dancing and screaming, attempting (unsuccessfully) to fly, and stabbing their dogs with forks just to name a few incidents.

Kids, just say no to being poisoned by *Claviceps purpurea*.

PROGNOSIS

First come the hallucinations, followed by twitching, muscle cramps, and the most intense sensation of pins and needles ever. You may feel insects crawling across your flesh. Then, bloodflow to your hands and feet is lost; it will feel as though your limbs have caught fire. This should last at least a few days. Your hands and feet will begin to rot and turn black. Eventually, they'll fall off, which doesn't mean you'll stop feeling like they're on fire. Most likely, when the hallucinations and pain end, you'll end up with a pretty bad case of brain damage.

PREVENTION

Claviceps purpurea is a parasite of rye. It grows particularly well on the grain during damp crop cycles and looks like tiny mushrooms. A trained eye will notice it immediately, and the crops can be destroyed before they do any damage. If, however, a trained eye is not available, the infected grain will go to the mill and be ground into infected flour, which will be sold to a baker who will make it into infected rye bread, which will be sold to a deli to be made into an infected roast-beef sandwich on rye with Dijon mustard and tomatoes, which you will eat, which will make you an infected person. To avoid ergotoxicosis, maybe order turkey on sourdough with mayonnaise and avocado (see eosinophilia-myalgia syndrome—page 123).

Infection by roast-beef sandwich is not very common these days. Much more common is infection through overuse of ergot-based drugs, such as methylergometrine, used to curb the effects of migraine headaches and control bleeding.

TREATMENT

Anticoagulant drugs and vasodilator drugs, such as dextran and hydralazine, respectively, may help curb the effects of ergotoxicosis. If they don't work, try taking sodium nitroprusside intravenously to relax the blood vessels and allow blood to flow more easily. Or just stick your arms and legs in a thresher and get it over with.

> ## Of Note . . .
>
> Ergotoxicosis has had a significant place throughout history. Great outbreaks spread throughout Europe during the Middle Ages, causing many to assume it was the wrath of God. In the eighteenth century, it crippled Peter the Great's army while en route to Constantinople to reclaim the city from the Turks. And many believe the disease may have been responsible for the erratic behavior that led to the Salem Witch Trials in the seventeenth century.

HYPONATREMIA
(ALSO WATER INTOXICATION)

In which you drink too much water and then fall into a coma and die.

SYMPTOMS

- fatigue
- apathy
- weakness
- cramping
- weight gain
- swelling
- nausea
- vomiting
- dizziness
- confusion
- headache
- disorientation
- fainting
- seizures
- coma

DIAGNOSIS

Remember how you've always been told that when you're running or doing something athletic you should be drinking lots of water to keep yourself hydrated? Well, forget that. No, you should still drink water. Just don't drink *too much* water. But don't drink *too little* water, either. What you should do actually, is drink *just the right amount* of water. In fact, you have to or you run the risk of collapsing and dying. What's the right amount? Who the hell knows? Everyone's different.

Everyone knows that drinking *too little* water will cause dehydration, which leads to dizziness, nausea, headaches, and, if it's particularly bad, death. But the new news is that drinking *too much* water will cause *hyponatremia* (hi''-po-nah-tre'-me-ah), which leads to dizziness, nausea, headaches, and, if it's particularly bad, death. Yes, the symptoms are exactly the same, and that can make things a little confusing while you're doubled over in pain and vomiting behind the basketball net, wondering what the hell you're supposed to do about it. But if you'd have just done what you were supposed to do in the first place and drank *just the right amount* of water, you wouldn't be in this situation.

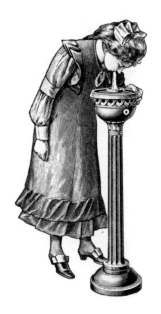

PROGNOSIS

Hyponatremia will come on very quickly, with symptoms gradually intensifying within an hour or so. As you sweat, your body expels water and sodium. Your body needs sodium to help it distribute water to all your muscles and organs. However, if you keep sweating out water and sodium and just replacing it with water, you'll have too much water and not enough sodium. Without that sodium to help distribute the water, the water's not getting put to any use and you start bloating. This is where the problems arise. You'll start to cramp and get nauseated. Water retention in your brain will make it actually begin swelling up inside your head. This will lead to headaches and seizures and coma and death, in that order.

And it all feels remarkably similar to dehydration.

PREVENTION

One surefire way to prevent hyponatremia is to make certain that, before you do anything particularly physical, you've taken in enough sodium into your diet. That way, as you drink *just the right amount* of water, you'll have enough sodium in your blood to keep the fragile water/sodium levels balanced.

However, don't add *too much* sodium to your diet, because that causes hypertension, which may lead to a heart attack and possibly death. What you should do is have *just the right amount* of sodium in your diet.

TREATMENT

If you begin to feel the symptoms of hyponatremia, stop whatever you're doing and eat something high in sodium; otherwise you'll run the risk of falling into a coma. Unless what you're actually feeling are the symptoms of dehydration (which are exactly the same), in which case you should stop whatever you're doing and drink plenty of water. But make sure the symptoms actually are those of dehydration, because if you only *think* it's dehydration but it's *really* hyponatremia and then you drink more water, you'll run the risk of falling into a coma.

> ## *Of Note . . .*
>
> Probably the best way to stave off hyponatremia is to never do anything remotely physical ever. Incidence of hyponatremia among people who sit around watching digital cable all day long is practically zero. However, too little physical activity causes coronary artery disease, which may lead to a heart attack and possibly death. What you need is *just the right amount* of physical activity.

TOXIC & FUNGAL

MUCORMYCOSIS
(ALSO ZYGOMYCOSIS)

In which you get a moldy brain.

SYMPTOMS

- fever
- sinus pain
- facial pain
- swelling
- headache
- labored breathing
- coughing up blood

- vision loss
- dilated pupils
- drooping eyelids
- bulging eyeballs
- blindness
- convulsions
- paralysis

DIAGNOSIS

There are acceptable places to find fungus, even if it's not always welcome. These include, but are not limited to: scenic forest paths, dilapidated shacks, between the tiles in your shower, and grilled portobello burgers with roasted red peppers. One place where it is definitely *not* acceptable to find fungus is on your brain. Your lungs, your eyes, your sinus cavity: also *not* acceptable.

In incidents of *mucormycosis* (mu''-kor-mi-ko'-sis), ordinary, run-of-the-mill fungus, such as can be found

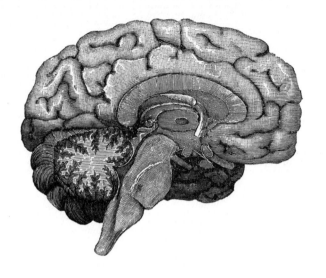

in soil or old vegetables, is inhaled as airborne spores. The fungus attaches itself to the soft tissue that lines the inside of your nose, mouth, or lungs and begins to multiply. Usually, your body's immune system will kill it off before any harm is done, but it may fight its way past, especially if your immune system has been compromised, such as by illness. If it manages to penetrate the soft tissue and invade your blood vessels, it will attempt to migrate toward your eyes and brain, causing inflammations that block the flow of blood, so that the body and brain begin to asphyxiate.

The fungus will also begin to destroy the tissue and bone with which it comes in contact, resulting in facial disfigurement or cavities in your lungs. It is possible to have mucormycosis destroy your skull from the inside out, causing your face to collapse in on itself.

PROGNOSIS

It's not looking good for you. There's about a 50 percent chance that you'll die within two weeks of the onset of symptoms, which is all the time the fungus needs to tear its way through your body, leaving cavities of dead flesh in its wake. Even if you do survive, you will most likely experience permanent residual effects such as blindness and brain damage. Mucormycosis is an aggressive disease, spreading quickly throughout the body, so if you think you might have it, don't waste any time. Begin panicking immediately.

> "It is possible to have mucormycosis destroy your skull from the inside out, causing your face to collapse in on itself."

Avoid at all costs: sugary foods, decaying plants, moldy food in the back of your refrigerator, manure, and common soil, as they may contain one of the four common types of fungus (mucor, rhizopus, rhizomucor, and absidia) that cause mucormycosis.

TREATMENT

You will have to have the infected tissue removed. It will all have to go. Even some tissue that has not been affected will have to go. Because the affected tissue does not bleed, many times doctors will just keep on cutting until the blood starts to flow. This is often quite disfiguring.

Of Note...

If you know someone with mucormycosis, and you're hoping to cheer him up, you should probably avoid telling any jokes that pun the word "fungi" with "fun guy." This is not because it is particularly offensive, but because that's just a bad joke.

TOXIC & FUNGAL

encephalitis

creutzfeldt-jakob disease

furious rabies

fatal familial insomnia

marburg hemorrhagic fever

VIRAL & PRIONIC

In which a free-roaming protein particle or a submicroscopic infective agent roams far and wide inside your body.

CREUTZFELDT–JAKOB DISEASE

In which your brain is eaten away by proteins until it resembles a sponge.

SYMPTOMS

- confusion
- memory loss
- loss of coordination
- involuntary muscle spasms
- itching
- paralysis
- mood swings
- depression
- impaired judgment
- degenerative eyesight
- insomnia
- dementia
- paranoia

DIAGNOSIS

Sometimes the phrase, "You have a brain like a sponge," is a compliment to your cognitive functions, meaning that you learn facts and skills quickly and easily; in much the same way that a sponge soaks up spilled pomegranate juice, you easily soak up any available information. However, if you have Creutzfeldt-Jakob disease, it means you literally have a brain like a sponge: porous and not very useful for retaining baseball statistics.

Creutzfeldt-Jakob disease (kroits'-felt yak'-ob) is caused by prions—transmissible, non-water-soluble proteins that get inside your brain, disrupting cell function and causing cell death. As the prions multiply exponentially, more and more of your cells begin to die, leaving little holes throughout your brain tissue. And thus, your brain ends up with the consistency of a sponge.

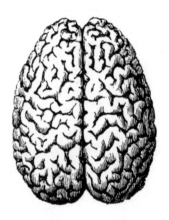

PROGNOSIS

You are going to die. There's no getting around it. The only questions are when, and how much pain and suffering will you and your family experience beforehand. At first, you will most likely experience some confusion and memory lapses, and then dementia, paranoia, and other forms of mental deterioration. This may be followed by phantom itching, a loss of motor function, spasms, and seizures. Your eyesight may be affected as you acquire blind spots and an inability to recognize shapes. Full-on paralysis may occur in the later stages. Eventually, you will fall into a coma. And then you will die. Death usually occurs within the two years after the initial onset of symptoms. Creutzfeldt-Jakob disease will occasionally cause alien hand syndrome (see page 74) and akinetic mutism (see page 70).

PREVENTION

Try not to get anything grafted onto your eyeball, spine, or brain, especially if that thing came from the cadaver of a person who had Creutzfeldt-Jakob disease. This will be a huge help in preventing Creutzfeldt-Jakob disease. Saying *thank you, but no* to having growth hormones injected into your person is probably also a good idea, as they are often taken from cadavers, any one of which may have been infected, even if they died before showing signs of the disease. There is also some speculation within the medical community that Creutzfeldt-Jakob disease may be transmissible through blood transfusions, so don't get any blood transfusions unless you really need them.

However, it is always possible that you could be carrying the seeds of Creutzfeldt-Jakob disease inside your genes right now—passed down from your parents or having just spontaneously appeared when you were conceived. There's no way to prevent that.

Although most victims of the disease are between the ages of fifty-seven and sixty-two, cases have occurred in people older than ninety and as young as seventeen. The first sign of symptoms has been known to occur up to a full thirty-eight years after the introduction of the disease into the body.

TREATMENT

There is no way to cure Creutzfeldt-Jakob disease. You may be able to get some doctors to inject pentosan polysulphate (a drug that mimics connective tissue) directly into your brain, though there is little evidence to suggest it will do any good.

Of Note . . .

Creutzfeldt-Jakob disease is a close relative of variant Creutzfeldt-Jakob disease, the human form of mad-cow disease, which is transferable through the consumption of infected meat, typically affects younger people, and inspired the 2003 production of *Mad Cow: The Musical*.

ENCEPHALITIS

In which your brain swells up inside your skull.

SYMPTOMS

- fever
- headache
- loss of appetite
- fatigue
- lethargy
- nausea
- vomiting
- stiff neck
- sensitivity to light
- different-sized pupils
- confusion
- disorientation
- personality changes
- seizures
- speech disturbance
- hearing loss
- hallucinations
- double vision
- loss of motor skills
- memory loss
- coma

DIAGNOSIS

Have you ever bashed your foot so bad that the skin beneath your ankle grew taut over blood-swelled muscle tissue and you could feel its flesh pressing tightly against the fabric of your shoe? Well, imagine that your foot is your brain and your shoe is your skull. That's encephalitis.

Encephalitis (en''-sef-ah-li'-tis) is an inflammation of the brain tissue. Your brain literally swells up inside your head, causing all sorts of bad things, like disorientation, speech impediments, hallucinations, seizures, loss of motor skills, and permanent brain damage. It occurs when a virus or bacterial infection in your body spreads to your brain.

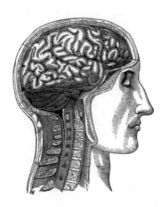

PROGNOSIS

If you get a particularly bad case of encephalitis, there's a decent chance you will die. However, assuming that you don't die, the pressure from your brain squeezing against the inside of your skull may cause permanent brain damage, resulting in memory loss, mental retardation, speech impediments, and loss of muscle control. Encephalitis has also been known to cause neurological diseases, such as akinetic mutism (page 70). If none of that happens, you will probably make a full recovery within a few months.

akinetic mutism (page 70)

VIRAL & PRIONIC

PREVENTION

There is no way to prevent encephalitis, per se. The only way to properly protect yourself from the disease is to protect yourself from all of the disorders that can trigger it. These include influenza, measles, rubella, mumps, shingles, mononucleosis, whooping cough, herpes simplex, HIV/AIDS, chicken pox, small pox, monkey pox, poliomyelitis, glandular fever, cryptococcosis, lymphocytic choriomeningitis, West Nile fever, cytomegalovirus, enteroviruses, listeriosis, lyssavirus, trichinosis, hepatitis, hypoglycemia, Epstein-Barr virus, varicella-zoster virus, dengue fever, Marburg hemorrhagic fever (page 198), Ebola, bacillary angiomatosis (page 40), and Toxoplasmosis[2], to name a few. If you keep yourself safe from those, you shouldn't have too much to worry about.

[2] Others disorders that can trigger encephalitis include, but are not limited to: Laryngotracheobronchitis Virus, Coital Exanthema Virus, Viral Diarrhea, Burkitt's Lymphoma, Cano Delgadito Virus, Kysanur Forest Disease, Warrego Virus, Caprine Arthritis Virus, Cassia Yellow Blotch, Kumba Virus, Colorado Tick Fever Virus, Buggy Creek Virus, Coxsackie Virus, European Swine Fever Virus, Yaba Virus, Bolivian Hemorrhagic Fever, Hemagglutinating Virus of Japan, Nelson Bay Virus, Abelson Leukemia Virus, Hirame Rhabdovirus, Junin Virus, Andean Potato Mottle Virus, Submaxillary Virus, Kemerovo Virus, Black Creek Canal Virus, Klamath Virus, O'Nyong-Nyong, Kyzylagach Virus, Swamp Fever, Neethling Virus, La Crosse Virus, Adelaide River Virus, Everglades Virus, Lymphocryptovirus, African Horse Sickness, Stomatitis Papulosa Virus, Spring Beauty Latent Virus, Camel Pox, Canary Pox, Capri Pox, Lepori Pox, Mollusci Pox, Psittacine Pox, Sheep Pox, Vole Pox, Aleutian Mink Disease Parvovirus, Mozambique Virus, Aujezky's Disease Virus, Muromegalovirus, Necrovirus, Newborn Pneumonitis Virus, Orf Virus, Phocine Distemper Virus, Kolongo Virus, Prospect Hill Virus, Bluetongue Virus, Puumala Virus, Ross River Virus, Semliki Forest Virus, Kilham's Rat Virus, Spumavirus, Yug Bogdanovac Virus, Mad Itch Virus, and Lumpy Skin Disease Virus.

Although several thousand cases of encephalitis are reported each year, it's suspected that many, many more go unreported.

TREATMENT

Get yourself to a hospital fast so they can monitor your vital signs and choose the proper course of medication to reduce the swelling and deal with the cause. If your brain is already too swelled up inside your head for you to think properly, ask a friend to take you to the hospital. It might be a good idea to ask a friend to be your encephalitis buddy now, so that if one of you ever feels your brain beginning to swell up, the other can be called on short notice and will be adequately prepared.

Of Note...

St. Louis encephalitis, the most popular form of the disease in the United States, is currently touring through more than forty states! Now you don't have to travel to the Show-Me State to get your brains on the mosquito-borne disease that infected 578 Missourians and killed 47 in 1975. An outbreak may be coming to your hometown! (Check the Centers for Disease Control and Prevention website for details. Not available in Alaska or Hawaii.)

FATAL FAMILIAL INSOMNIA

In which you never sleep again.

SYMPTOMS

- insomnia
- dementia
- loss of motor skills
- numbness
- lack of tears
- panic attacks

- agitation
- hallucinations
- skin discoloration
- phobias
- incontinence
- loss of speech

DIAGNOSIS

Fatal familial insomnia is a prion disease, related to Creutzfeldt-Jakob disease (page 182), in which rogue proteins turn your brain into a sponge. However, in this case, the part of your brain that is affected is the thalamus, which controls your ability to sleep. You actually lose the ability to sleep, and since your body cannot function without sleep, it starts to fall apart. And then you die.

Because this disease is inherited, it can be traced through lineages. If a relative, such as your grandfather or aunt, died of fatal familial insomnia, there's a pretty decent

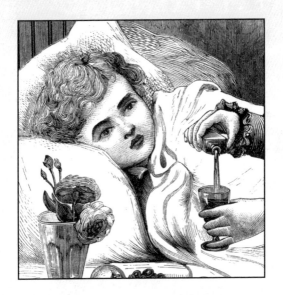

chance that you will as well. And you'll be fully aware of that. What this means is that every time you lie awake in bed, unable to sleep, you'll have to wonder if your possibly-run-of-the-mill insomnia represents an early stage of the disease. Of course, thinking along those lines won't help you get to sleep any faster. The more time you lie awake worrying if you have the disease, the more you'll become convinced that you have the disease, even if you don't.

Most people who have fatal familial insomnia begin seeing signs in their late forties or early fifties, but it has struck people in their thirties and sixties. Because the disease usually pops up after a person's child-rearing

years, if you think you may be carrying the disease, you will
have to make a choice: either have children, knowing that
you may be cursing them with this nightmare, or don't have
children and then possibly discover that you didn't have the
disease after all.

PROGNOSIS

You will definitely die, most likely within a year of the onset
of symptoms. On the bright side, since you won't be sleeping
through most of that year, it will feel like an eternity.

During the first few months, you will experience some
insomnia along with panic attacks and strange phobias,
such as being afraid of not being able to fall asleep (actually,
that's not so strange, I guess). Then come the hallucinations: Perhaps you'll see anthropomorphic mice climbing
out of the walls to mock you in their nightcaps and dressing
gowns. After that comes total insomnia. One day, you wake
up, and that's the last time you ever do that. Your body begins to whither; your brain becomes so exhausted that you
slip into total dementia, wandering around your house in a
half-dream state, swatting at buzzing bottle-fly alarm clocks
that don't exist. Then you slip into a coma. And then you
die. Luckily, by this point, death is probably welcomed.

PREVENTION

Try not to be related to any of your relatives who might be carrying the disease.

TREATMENT

The disease can be easily cured with aspirin and warm milk. Wouldn't that be nice? Unfortunately, it's not true. There is no cure. Even sleeping pills are useless. Some scientists think that the disease can be cured through gene therapy, in which a non-corrupted gene is inserted into the thalamus, altering your genetic expression. But that most likely won't be available for another ten or fifteen years. That's if it even works at all.

Of Note...

Fatal familial insomnia is closely related to sporadic fatal insomnia. In fact, it's exactly the same. Except that sporadic fatal insomnia is not genetic and just happens to regular people for no apparent reason, leaving victims with no one to blame. So, see, it could be worse.

VIRAL & PRIONIC

FURIOUS RABIES
(ALSO HYDROPHOBIA)

In which you become crazed, violent, and mortally afraid of water.

SYMPTOMS

- itching
- headache
- fever
- chills
- fatigue
- nausea
- vomiting
- sore throat
- loss of appetite
- irritability
- stiff muscles
- pupil dilation
- increased salivation
- foaming at the mouth
- drooling
- fear of water

- depression
- restlessness
- insomnia
- sensitivity to sound
- sensitivity to light
- sensitivity to temperature
- mania
- barking
- biting
- muscle spasms
- throat spasms
- difficulty swallowing
- difficulty breathing
- convulsions
- paralysis
- coma

You will find that few social faux pas will cause the invitations for garden soirées to dry up faster than showing up with an advanced case of furious rabies. With that in mind, please consider the following:

DO remember to say, "Thank you, but no" if offered an unwanted glass of Pellegrino.
DON'T scream wildly, knock the offending beverage to the ground, and lunge at the valet's throat with fingers curled into claws.

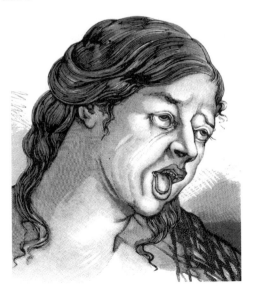

DO engage in witty banter about current events with other guests in attendence.

DON'T jump onto the lawn furniture and bark furiously, while saliva foams around the corners of your lips.

DO compliment your host on his or her choice of savory smoked game hors d'oeuvres provided for your pleasure.

DON'T attempt to bite your host on the face.

PROGNOSIS

The virus *Rhabdoviridae* (rab"do-vir'-i-de) will initially cause flu-like symptoms, such as fever and nausea, for several days. This is followed by anxiety, depression, and insomnia. This will progress to furious rabies, in which you become manic and prone to fits of irrational violence, such as biting and clawing. The act of swallowing will cause spasms in the throat, so you will learn to fear water, screaming at the sight of it. Unwilling to swallow your own saliva, it will drip from your mouth or foam around your lips. Your muscles will gradually become paralyzed, and you will fall into a coma. Then you will die.

PREVENTION

The rabies virus is transmitted through saliva, usually via an animal (or human) bite, such as a wild raccoon or a bat, so be very careful when outdoors. These animals are crazy and highly infectious. And they're waiting for you.

TREATMENT

The rabies virus is very slow-moving, with symptoms not becoming apparent for several months after infection. Once symptoms arise, it is almost certainly fatal, but you should have plenty of time to get the rabies vaccine injected into you after the virus is introduced into your body. That is assuming that you realize that you have been infected.

Of Note . . .

To date, there have only been ten reported cases of people surviving infection of the *Rhabdoviridae* virus once the symptoms presented themselves, and four of those cases were completely fabricated by the author to make the situation seem slightly less dire.

VIRAL & PRIONIC

MARBURG HEMORRHAGIC FEVER

In which you are infected by a virus, your body falls apart, and then you die, all within the span of about two weeks.

SYMPTOMS

- fever
- chills
- headache
- nausea
- vomiting
- confusion
- incoherence
- memory loss
- hallucinations
- loss of appetite
- weight loss

- lethargy
- muscle pain
- abdominal pain
- chest pain
- sore throat
- itching
- rash
- diarrhea
- bleeding from the nose and/or gums

DIAGNOSIS

Do not mess around with Marburg hemorrhagic fever. If your friend or loved one tells you that he or she has Marburg hemorrhagic fever, leave. Get the hell out of there. Get in a car and drive someplace far away from that person. If an outbreak of Marburg hemorrhagic fever occurs in your hometown, get on a plane and fly someplace far away from that town (unless you have already been infected with the disease without knowing it, in which case you'd be helping to spread Marburg hemorrhagic fever on to other unsuspecting people and towns).

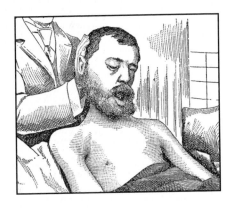

Marburg hemorrhagic fever (mar'-berg hem''-o-raj'-ik fe'-ver) is a severe infectious *Filoviridae* virus (the only other *Filoviridae* viruses are the four types of ebola, which you should also not mess with), which is capable of being passed from person to person at such a rate that outbreaks can quickly cripple entire communities. In March 2005, an outbreak of Marburg hemorrhagic fever ripped itself through the small African state of Angola, and in less than one month's time, 266 cases of the disease were reported, and 244 resulted in death. Once the virus attaches itself to a living human cell, it kills that cell and then uses it to make more microscopic killing machines to go off and attach themselves to more living human cells, until you are dead.

To summarize: Do not mess around with Marburg hemorrhagic fever.

PROGNOSIS

There's a very good chance that you're going to die. Various outbreaks have had differing mortality rates. The Angola outbreak had a mortality rate greater than 90 percent, and a similar outbreak in the Democratic Republic of Congo had a mortality rate of 83 percent.

After anywhere from five to ten days following infection, the disease's effects will hit you quickly and harshly. You can expect fever, chills, headache, and muscle aches. Five days later comes the rash, a spotted, bumpy, discolored patch that spreads across your chest, back, and stomach. And then nausea, chest and abdominal pain, sore throat, and diarrhea set in, followed by oral and nasal hemorrhaging, jaundice, inflammation of the pancreas, severe weight loss, delirium, shock, liver failure, and multi-organ dysfunction. When death finally comes, about a week after the onset of symptoms, you'll most likely be grateful.

PREVENTION

Do not engage in any physical contact with anybody who may have engaged in any physical contact, within the past ten days, with anybody who may have engaged in any physical contact with anybody who may have had Marburg hemorrhagic fever.

TREATMENT

There is no known treatment specifically for Marburg hemorrhagic fever. However, hospital therapy, such as having your electrolytes monitored and having lost blood replaced, will improve your chances for survival to some degree.

Of Note . . .

The first people known to be infected with Marburg hemorrhagic fever were laboratory researchers in Germany and Yugoslavia in 1967. The disease was passed on to them by African green monkeys, imported for research in the preparation of a polio vaccine. The monkeys were very cute, until they died.

VIRAL & PRIONIC

ACKNOWLEDGMENTS

I would sincerely like to thank...

Adrienne Wiley, Avra Romanowitz, Rachel E. Devitt, everyone at becker&mayer!, and...

...Nelly Reifler, and...

.:.Michael J. Ewing, Jennifer Toner, Jason Toogood, Jessica Wyant, Jack Pope, Clay Cansler, Upma Singh, Michelle McCormick, Michael Cannon, Chris Welsh, Joe Morris, Lara Manogg, James Stevens, Danielle Tersigni, Tricia Mueller, Nick Henderson, Nick Battiste, Bob Toogood, Michael Collins, Bernadette Toner, Rick Horner, Tony DiGerolamo, Jon Sales, Phil George, Micah Best, John Boggi, Brian Holcomb, Michelle Budenz, Patrick Hauth, Tara Murtha, and...

...Tom Hartman, Rose Gowen, Matthew Tobey, Josh Abraham, Geoff Wolinetz, Nick Jezarian, Maud Newton, Heather Kelley, Michael Hearst, Christopher Monks, Darci Ratliff, Leonard Kelly, Patrick Knowles, Bob Hasegawa, J. Edward Keyes, Lee Klein, Pitchaya Sudbanthad, Shauna McKenna, Gina Zucker, Peter Dabbene, Julia Chang, Duane Swierczynski, and...

...The Cabal, The Waitstaff, Hypnotoad, and...

...Kim Murphy, Jill Day, everyone at Elsevier, and...

...Susan DiClaudio, Dennis DiClaudio, Denelle DiClaudio, Anthony DiClaudio, Diandra DiClaudio, Carmen Panarello, Anthony DiMaggio, Ray DiClaudio, my entire family, and...

...a thousand other people I wish I had the space to list here; I would happily step in front of an infected mosquito for any one of them.

I would also like acknowledge...

...The Centers for Disease Control and Prevention, The World Health Organization, The Straight Dope, and eMedicine.

INDEX OF SYMPTOMS